This essential, in-depth  purpose of accelerating Based on Ganga and Ta the wisdom lineage of t offerings are as applicable in our postmodern times as they were 5000 years ago. I highly recommend this healing and nourishing book.

– **Michael Bernard Beckwith**
Author of *Spiritual Liberation* and *Life Visioning*

Herbs for Spiritual Development is a gentle and eloquent narrative about the power of Tonic Herbs for healing, radiant health, and spiritual evolution. It is wonderful that Ganga and Tara have established the deepest goal of using Tonic Herbs to enhance spiritual attainment. This is, as they stated, the point of longevity. These Tonic Herbs also help us harmonize back to the natural and cosmic laws that our world society has abandoned. Another major teaching they share is that one cannot "herbalize" their way to enlightenment and we also need to do energizing movement, breath, and meditation as part of a full holistic liberation approach. The use of these Tonic Herbs with live-foods (perhaps what the Taoist masters lived on before going to only Tonic Herbs) is my suggested optimal diet for spiritual nutrition and the way I've been living for years. The journey shared in this book is their living of the Three Treasures in a gentle and joyous way. I highly recommend this book, not only for beginners in Tonic Herbalism, but also as a reminder to all about the larger meaning of the use of Tonic Herbs.

– **Gabriel Cousens, M.D.,** Yogi in the Siddha Lineage

To become what the Daoist masters call a Flying Immortal, it is important to work on one's spiritual, mental, as well as nutritional intake. The tonic herbs lovingly described here have been used for centuries by those aspirants wishing to perfect their human vehicles for higher attainment.

– **Peter Mt. Shasta,** Author of *Apprentice to the Masters: Adventures of a Western Mystic, Book II*

Herbs for Spiritual Development by Ganga and Tara is a delightful guide, full of important information for those of us who want to enjoy Tonic Herbs and spiritual growth. Ron Teeguarden is a teacher and a dear friend of mine who I like to call the "American Lao Tzu." He has the energy of a very old ginseng root to help people live a healthy and happy life through natural herbs and Taoist teaching. I became a monk at the Shaolin Temple in China when I was eight years old and underwent intensive training in martial arts there for eleven years. The Chinese Tonic Herbs have been used at the Shaolin Temple for centuries to improve health, enhance athletic performance and promote spiritual development.

– *Wang Bo*, Shaolin 34th Generation Warrior Monk and Founder of Hungrymonk Yoga

This profound book sends before it "a call." It called to me from the moment I heard of its existence. I could feel the very fire of Life that commands change. I could feel the ancient herbs calling to me. The book carries an unspeakable energy. It is a call to humanity to align mind, body, and spirit. It is a call to align with Wholeness, the Truth of our Being. This book has the power behind it to change the course of humanity. It has the power to help build a numinous culture of balance. I am in deep appreciation to Ganga and Tara and Ron Teeguarden for being wayshowers in the West, sending forth this Consciousness of these holy herbs to be shared. It is Time! And I add…that in taking these tonic essence herbs, I am feeling a calmness that I simply did not know that I did not have!

– *Mary Saint-Marie*, Mystic Artist, Writer, and Spiritual Educator

In their book, *Herbs For Spiritual Development*, Ganga and Tara truly took me on an exciting adventure through the world of Tonic Herbs. Ganga and Tara's Journey took them to China to Sacred Mountains and Lakes where very pure Herbal plants are grown in pristine soil. The photography of China's sacred places is exquisite. Part Two of the book delves into 22 Tonic Herbs, with beautiful photographs of each herb, the type of nourishment the Herb gives the body, and the Spiritual Qualities of that Herb. Their adventure captivated my attention and brought me to a sacred space within to really appreciate the Herbs. I now feel a deep connection with the Tonic Herbs and the Sacred Tea Ceremony. The Tonic Herbs are part of my daily, sacred prayers. I love this book for the way it opened my life to a new world of using Tonic Herbs, Elixirs, and Teas for longevity.

– *Violet Schindler*, Mystic Storyteller

Herbs for Spiritual Development

*Ganga's Adventures
in the World of Tonic Herbs*

by Ganga and Tara

Preface by Ron Teeguarden

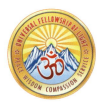

Universal Fellowship of Light Publishing
2017

Herbs for Spiritual Development

Ganga's Adventures in the World of Tonic Herbs

Copyright © 2017 by Universal Fellowship of Light Publishing
All rights reserved.

No portion of this book, except for brief review, may be reproduced, stored in a retrieval system, or transmitted in any form or by any means—electronic, mechanical, photocopying, recording, or otherwise—without written permission of the publisher. For information contact Universal Fellowship of Light Publishing.

Universal Fellowship of Light Publishing
P.O. Box 803
Mt. Shasta, CA 96067
Visit our website at www.universalfellowshipoflight.com

ISBN-13: 978-0-9983726-0-0
ISBN-10: 0-9983726-0-9

The information presented in this book is derived from traditional and modern texts and from oral teachings reflecting the observations of numerous authorities on Chinese herbs. This information should not be used to diagnose, treat, or attempt to prevent any disease without the advice of a qualified physician familiar with your medical history and condition, as well as a qualified health practitioner knowledgeable about Chinese herbs. The Chinese Tonic Herbs are traditionally used to promote health, not counteract disease. If you are suffering from any ailment that may require medical attention, do not consume herbs unless advised to do so by a physician.

Front cover art by Ganga
Front cover design by Ganga and Baruch Inbar
Photo on page 5 provided by Ron Teeguarden, All Rights Reserved
Illustration on page 24 by Tara
Index created by Kenneth Hassman
Printed in Hungary

HERBS FOR SPIRITUAL DEVELOPMENT is sponsored by the Universal Fellowship of Light, the goal of which is to promote the health of body, mind, and spirit and assist in the enlightenment of humanity.

DEDICATION

This book is dedicated
with deepest love and respect
to our Daoist Herbal Master,
Dan-O Sun Sha (Ron Teeguarden),

to his Daoist teacher Master Sung Jin Park,

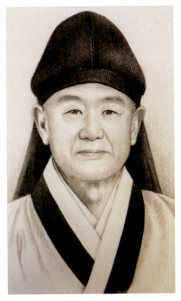

Master Sung Jin Park

to his teacher Moo San Do Sha,

and to the lineage of Daoist Herbal Masters
throughout the ages.

PART ONE

GANGA'S ADVENTURES IN THE WORLD OF TONIC HERBS

1. A Door Opens 3
2. The Apprenticeship Begins 8
3. How Ron Teeguarden Discovered Tonic Herbs 12
4. Tonic Herbalism Takes Root In America 14
5. The Three Treasures Philosophy 18
6. The History of Chinese Herbalism 22
7. Daoist Mountain Hermits—Living in Harmony with Nature . 25
8. Daoist Longevity Techniques 27
9. The Best of the Ancient and Modern 32
10. Becoming a Tea Master 34
11. The First Night in Beijing—Seeing the Goji Lady 38
12. A Chinese Herb Market 43
13. Di Dao 46
14. Expedition to Changbai Mountain 48
15. Encounters with Notable People 53
16. Seven Years in India 59
17. Masters of Longevity 62
18. Returning to China with Ron and Yanlin 66
19. Pilgrimage to the Shaolin Temple 70
20. The Secrets of Spiritual Development 81
21. How to Take Tonic Herbs 85
22. Making It Easier for You to Start Receiving the Benefits 88

PART TWO

22 TONIC HERBS BY TARA

1. Reishi 91
2. Schizandra Berries 97
3. Ginseng 101
4. Siberian Ginseng 107
5. American Ginseng 111
6. Gynostemma 113
7. Rhodiola 117
8. Cordyceps 121
9. Polygonum 125
10. Rehmannia Root 129
11. Chaga 131
12. Lycium Fruit 135
13. Astragalus 139
14. Albizzia 143
15. Wild Asparagus Root 145
16. Polygala Root 149
17. Spirit Poria 153
18. Pearl 157
19. Zizyphus Seed 161
20. Dendrobium 165
21. Eucommia Bark 169
22. Snow Lotus 173

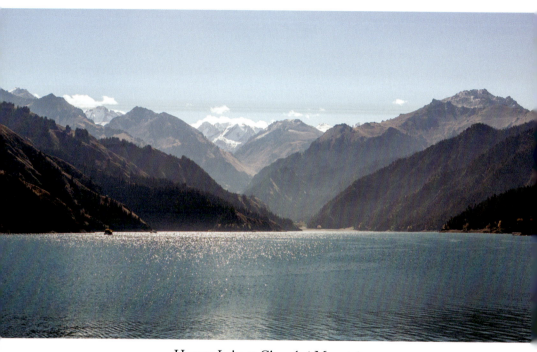

Heaven Lake at Changbai Mountain

PREFACE

Ganga Nath has been my friend for two decades. It's odd to call a man of such accomplishment my apprentice, but that is how it worked out for the first few years of our relationship. At the time, my wife Yanlin and I operated an herbal realm from a sprawling house in west Los Angeles, and I maintained a range of apprentices for several years there. Ganga, who was known as Kris Kane at the time, was the only one who we invited to live with us, which he did, and he lived and breathed herbs every day of his life for those years. We made custom teas with a wonderful clinical extraction apparatus (tanks and extractors), very largely for celebrities, as it turned out. The clients literally visited us from all over the world every day.

Ganga served as my "elixir-maker" for more than two years, handling extraordinary herbs and extraordinary requests for extraordinary people on all kinds of paths. We served an ex-president, some of the biggest television and movie stars in the world, some of music's most iconic figures, artists and moguls, young and old, men and women from every culture you can imagine. It makes me laugh and smile thinking about the range of characters we served! Ganga made precision elixirs based on the recipes I wrote up for each of these clients.

Ganga, being the wonderful human being that he is, served with amazing grace, skill, focus, and love. Our clients loved to visit with him. He had long since become an evolved human and his interest was in transforming himself and our clients. He was perceived as a mentor by most of these people—who were themselves very accomplished. It was a remarkable period.

I taught him as much as I could in those years. In the late 1990s we started having Ganga travel with us to China as our photographer, a skill in which he is proficient. He documented our trip to Changbai Mountain, to the Reishi Mushroom and Ginseng farms, to the Schizandra forests, to exotic tea shops, and more. I am sure that these excursions benefited his "feeling" for the world of tonic herbalism, the most evolved herbal system in the world.

Tonic Herbs are the special class of herbs that promote human glowing health by providing life force derived from the earth and sky by these remarkable plants. The "tonic" system was developed in Asia nearly three thousand years ago and remains the most widely used herbal system on earth. Ganga, the great teacher that he is, explains the system and the herbs in this book. He also paints a picture of how these herbs affected him and his approach to life.

Eventually, Ganga left my immediate sphere and spent time teaching and studying elsewhere. India called. He spent many years in India, practicing his "yoga" at a high level with enlightened gurus—this is when he became "Ganga." Before he worked with me he had sat at the very side of the illustrious Maharishi Mahesh Yogi, the guru of the Beatles, Donovan, and others in the 1960s, and the founder of Transcendental Meditation.

It is an honor to me that Ganga Nath has decided to write this memoir of the period when we worked together. It was a wonderful, alchemical, and transformational time and space. I hope his story induces many more people to explore the world of Tonic Herbs, the Daoist art of life cultivation, and the path of glowing health, which is a path of wisdom. I know it will provide you with a view of a brilliant man, who with the help and love of his wife Tara, is serving humanity by shedding spiritual light everywhere he passes and beyond.

Blessings to you all,

Ron Teeguarden, Dan-O Sun Sha, Master Herbalist, and Daoist Master of Kook Sun Do

INTRODUCTION

When I met Ron Teeguarden, I had already been deeply involved in the spiritual path for over forty years. I had taught meditation for over 30 years, started Dharma centers both in America and Europe, and run a one hundred acre retreat center. During that time, I was fortunate to study with some of the greatest living spiritual teachers from a variety of spiritual traditions: Hindu, Buddhist, Sufi, Tibetan Buddhist, and Zen.

One of my first spiritual teachers was Maharishi Mahesh Yogi. Maharishi once said that there are three things that are most important to know about in life: mantras, gems, and herbs. While I knew a lot of mantras and something about gems, when I met Ron Teeguarden, I knew next to nothing about herbs. That was about to change on the day that I met Ron and became his apprentice.

In the first few moments that I met Ron, he started teaching me about what Tonic Herbs are and how they have been used by Daoist and Buddhist sages for thousands of years to promote health, longevity, and enlightenment. I already understood the value of learning from a master who is part of an authentic lineage. So it appealed to me that Ron was a Master Daoist Herbalist and that he had learned about the Tonic Herbs from his Korean Daoist Master, Sung Jin Park. The paramount interest in my life was the attainment of enlightenment, and if Tonic Herbs could assist me in attaining enlightenment, then I wanted to learn everything I could about them.

As my apprenticeship with Ron continued, I began to understand why the Daoist and Buddhist sages were also herbal masters. They understood the mind/body connection and knew that the health of the body plays a major role in developing consciousness. Furthermore, these great sages possessed a deep knowledge of the subtle energy channels within the human being, and they understood how the Tonic Herbs contribute to the evolution of consciousness. They also valued longevity, because the longer you live the greater the chances are that you will attain enlightenment. In my over forty years on the spiritual path, I had already learned that to be born as a human being with the chance to become enlightened is a precious opportunity, not to be squandered. I was determined to learn all I could from Ron Teeguarden, who I respected as a living custodian of one of the most profound wisdom traditions on Earth.

The three years that I lived with Ron and his family was one of the greatest blessings of my life. Traditionally, in ancient times, one lived with one's herbal master and observed how they lived each day. The transmission of wisdom was not book-learned but was often absorbed non-verbally.

I am deeply grateful to Ron for his generosity and patience with me. He is widely considered to be the Father of Chinese Tonic Herbalism in America. Somehow I was blessed with the opportunity of a lifetime to live with him and his family and to learn a small portion of his vast understanding of Tonic Herbalism.

The great Buddhist and Daoist herbal masters are true treasures of humanity. They possess a time-tested ancient body of knowledge that can assist those of us living in the modern world to live happy, healthy, and fulfilled lives. It is my pleasure to play a small role in communicating this ancient Art of Living by recounting my experiences living and apprenticing with a Daoist Herbal Master.

Ganga Nath
Mount Shasta, California
November 11, 2016

GANGA'S ADVENTURES IN THE WORLD OF TONIC HERBS

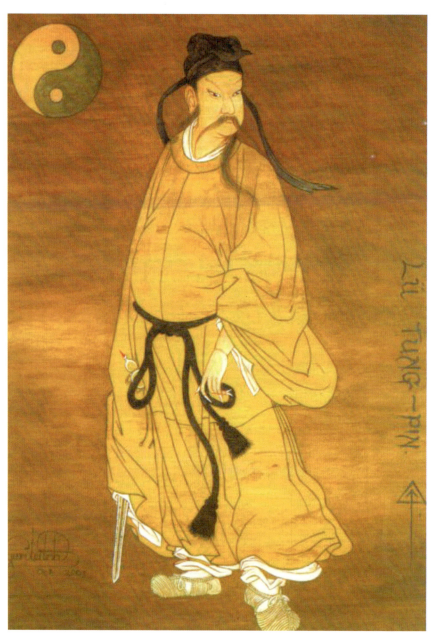

Ancestor Lu said: "If you want to learn the Great Way, you must value the Three Treasures. Without the Three Treasures you cannot live long, and deep attainment cannot be reached in the limited time we have. So without knowing and valuing the Three Treasures you will not learn the Great Way."

1. A DOOR OPENS

There are moments in one's life when a door opens, often unexpectedly, and one is introduced to a whole new dimension of one's existence. After that, life is never the same again. New horizons open before you, new possibilities are presented, new truths are fathomed, and new realizations are comprehended. I was blessed with such a life-expanding experience on a fine day in June of 1997.

I was visiting a friend in Los Angeles, and one day, feeling bored, I looked in my phone book for any old friends who might still be living in Los Angeles. I found the phone number of a friend who I'd taught meditation with back in New York in the 1970s. I hadn't seen him in about twenty years, and I thought it would be great to renew our friendship. When I reached him on the phone, he invited me to join him for dinner at his favorite Italian restaurant. Over a delicious meal, we caught up on all that had transpired in our lives since we last saw each other. As we finished eating, he looked me in the eyes and said, "There's someone you should meet. I'm not going to tell you anything about him, except his first name, which is Ron." Needless to say, he had aroused my curiosity. Taking out a pen, he began writing on the back of a business card and said, "This is his phone number. Call him tomorrow and tell him that I said that you two should meet." As I drove away, I wondered who this "Ron" could possibly be and why my friend felt that it was so important that we should meet.

When I woke up the next morning, I found the business card in my pocket and called the phone number written on the back. When someone answered the phone, I asked, "Are you Ron?" He replied, "Yes." I told him that my friend had suggested that we meet and he replied, "Come on over," and gave me his address. A few moments later, I was driving to Brentwood, an upscale area of Los Angeles just west of Beverly Hills. Little did I know how my life was about to change and what an amazing spiritual adventure awaited me.

I pulled up in front of a wood-shingled house that looked relatively modest, considering that the area is where many movie stars and famous people live. As I approached the front door, I noticed two unusual things that were the first indications that I was entering a magical space. To the left of the front door was a beautiful sculpture made from a tree trunk with the Daoist Immortals carved in it. To the right of the door there was a broom that you might find a monk sweeping with in a Zen monastery. I rang the doorbell, eager to discover what lay inside.

The door opened and I was greeted by a friendly tall man with an imposing presence who invited me inside. Right away, I noticed to my right a towering wood sculpture of a Buddha. I followed the person I only knew as "Ron" as he made his way down the hall and turned into the living room. As I looked around the room, I immediately felt that I was no longer in Los Angeles, or even America. I had somehow been transported to ancient China. The room was exquisitely decorated with Chinese art. The chairs were massive, formed from the roots of trees, and the counters were carved from tree trunks. Along one entire wall were shelves of wooden drawers with Chinese characters painted on them. I was awestruck and asked, "What do you do?" Ron explained that he was a Chinese Tonic Herbalist and this was his herbarium.

Now, I have to explain that at that point I knew practically nothing about herbs. I think that the only herbs I knew anything about were Ginseng and Echinacea. Probably noticing the puzzled look on my face, Ron began to explain what Chinese Tonic Herbalism is. He started by taking me around the room and using the art on the walls to explain certain basic principles of Tonic Herbalism. He began with a painting that depicted the Chinese conception of heaven. In the center of heaven was a stone pedestal, and on top of the pedestal was a mushroom. He explained that this was a Reishi Mushroom and that it was considered the King of all Chinese herbs. He handed me a Reishi Mushroom and explained that another name for it in China is the Mushroom of Immortality and Good Fortune. I had never seen a mushroom like this. Instead of being soft and squishy, it was hard like wood and had a beautiful orangish-red luster.

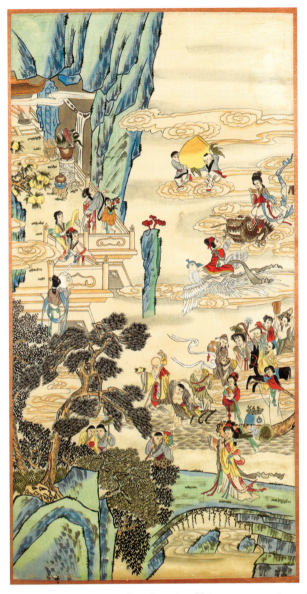

A Reishi Mushroom sits on a pedestal in the Chinese conception of Heaven.
(Photo courtesy of Ron Teeguarden)

As I held this large exotic mushroom in my hand, Ron continued to give me a tour of the herbarium. Next, he pointed out a painting of a beautiful fair-skinned maiden, dressed in flowing robes, carrying in her hand a Reishi Mushroom. Ron explained that this was the Goddess Magu, who the Chinese believe brought the Reishi

Mushroom down from Heaven to Earth for mankind. Then, he took me through a hallway lined with plastic bins containing the highest quality Tonic Herbs in the world. He explained that he went on expeditions to China to gather these herbs and that he was always searching for higher and higher quality herbs. After opening several containers to let me savor their aroma, he took me into a room that contained a very large machine that was used to brew teas extracted from the Tonic Herbs. He showed me how several pounds of raw herbs were placed in a canvas bag, and then the bag was lowered into a very large pressure cooker filled with filtered water. After the herbs had cooked for about an hour, a valve was switched and the boiling tea flowed into a bagging machine that sealed the tea into high-quality plastic pouches. Ron explained that these were custom teas personally made and shipped to his clients around the world.

Leading me back into the living room, Ron continued to explain what makes Chinese Tonic Herbalism unique. He said that over thousands of years the Chinese have developed the most sophisticated knowledge of herbs of any culture on Earth. He explained that the Chinese have researched and documented the effects of many hundreds of herbs. He said that the Tonic Herbs are a small subset of all the herbs and that they are called the Superior Herbs because they have no negative side-effects and can be consumed every day of one's life. The other herbs are medicinal herbs and can be used for shorter periods of time. The medicinal herbs are called the Inferior Herbs, not because they are bad, but because they are used to cure disease, whereas the Tonic Herbs are used to develop such a state of Radiant Health that one does not become ill in the first place. In ancient China, you paid the doctor to keep you healthy, not to cure you when you became sick.

As Ron continued to explain how the Tonic Herbs were adaptogenic, helping your body to maintain a state of balance, I began to understand that this was an ancient and profound science of preventive medicine. A light was beginning to dawn. I felt a deep affinity with this place that I had somehow been drawn to. It was like my inner being resonated with the aesthetics of the room and the potent herbs within it. But, beyond the externals, I felt an inner familiarity with

Ron, almost like he was an old friend from long ago. Feeling a bit dazzled, I looked around the room, taking in all its beauty, and said, "I would love to live in a house like this." Ron looked at me and said, "Would you?" I repeated, "Yes, I would really love to live in a place like this." He said, "Would you like to live here?" Feeling a bit confused, I asked, "Are you asking me if I want to live in your house?" To my amazement, he replied, "Yes, there's an empty apartment in the back. You can move in and be my apprentice." To say that I was shocked is to put it mildly. I'd only known this person for less than thirty minutes, and I knew nothing about herbs. I was an herbal virgin, living in Chicago, with no plan to move to Los Angeles. Now, I was being offered the opportunity to move into the home of a Master Daoist Herbalist who I barely knew and become his apprentice. I thought about it for about ten seconds and said, "I'd love to!"

It was a magical moment. It wasn't a hard decision. My inner being felt with certainty that a door had opened and that through this door a myriad of wonders awaited me. There was nothing to think about, no reason to weigh options or to consider the many implications of the decision. The answer within was pure and simple, "Walk through," and I did.

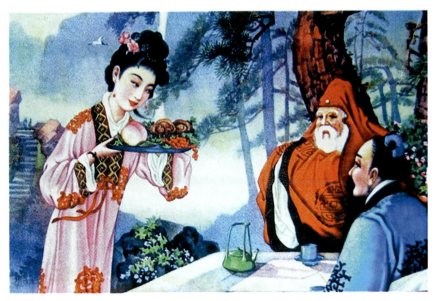

The Goddess Magu offering Tonic Herbs to a Daoist Master and his disciple

2. THE APPRENTICESHIP BEGINS

Now that I'd taken the leap of faith, there were some practical issues to consider, like how I was going to move to Los Angeles. I had been living in an apartment right on the Chicago River in the heart of downtown Chicago. I had recently taken my eight-year-old cousin to Germany to see her favorite singer Jewel perform in Berlin, and then I had immediately gone to the Hopi reservation to photograph Chief Dan Evehema, the oldest living Keeper of the Hopi Prophesies. Chief Dan was 106 at the time, and I photographed him crawling on his hands and knees among the corn that is sacred to the Hopi. I felt extremely blessed to meet this wise elder and was fortunate to meet Chief Dan when I did, because he passed away shortly thereafter. The cost of traveling to Germany, Arizona, and Los Angeles had left me in a tenuous financial situation, so I wondered how I was going to rent a truck to move to Los Angeles. Ron, out of the kindness of his heart, offered to pay for the rental of the truck and the gas.

As I left Chicago and drove across America on Route 66, heading for sunny Southern California, I thought about how my life had taken this sudden turn, and I marveled at the series of events that were leading me onward into the unknown. When I arrived at Ron's house, he told me to make myself comfortable in the apartment in the rear of the house. Ron suggested that I get a good night's sleep and said we'd talk in the morning. As I fell asleep, I marveled over the fact that I was now living in a Master Herbalist's home. The excitement was mixed with a slight nervousness which was the result of worrying over whether I would be up to the challenge of being the apprentice of a Master Herbalist. I wondered what would be expected of me and whether I would be able to succeed in the training. Only time would tell. I let go of all worry and trusted that the same force that had brought me here would guide me on my path.

The next morning, I showered, meditated, got dressed, and went down the hall to the living room. As I opened the door and stepped into the living room, who did I see but one of the most famous actresses in the world, waiting for her consultation with Ron. When she left, another A-list movie star arrived for her appointment with Ron. Then, one of the most popular current singers arrived for his appointment. This continued all day long. It was a constant stream of the world's most famous actors, musicians, and singers. Many of these people had been clients of Ron ever since he first had a small herb store on Abbot Kinney Boulevard in Venice, California. They came to him because the Tonic Herbs improved their health and helped them maintain a sense of centeredness in the hectic life of Hollywood.

At first I was star-struck, seeing these celebrities up close, but soon I discovered that, although they had achieved great fame and fortune, they had all the same problems of ordinary people. As time went by, I came to see fame as more of a curse than a blessing. One of the highest-paid actors in Hollywood told me one day that he woke up each day wanting to kill himself. Many of these celebrities, who people idolize, suffered from anxiety, depression, chronic fatigue, physical pains, and emotional problems, just like ordinary people, and they found that the Tonic Herbs helped them lead active, creative, and fulfilled lives.

I knew from my childhood that money doesn't make you happy. I was fortunate to grow up in one of the wealthiest communities in America and went to an exclusive private school for boys. My childhood friends' families were some the wealthiest people in America. Their fathers were CEOs of companies. Their grandfathers had founded major corporations. These were the people that most people believe are the lucky ones, but at an early age I discovered that the problems that plague ordinary people were theirs as well. When I saw alcoholic fathers cheating on their wives, mothers addicted to Valium, and their sons becoming alcoholics in high school, I decided that although money was useful in life, it certainly didn't provide true happiness.

That was when I turned toward the East in search of where the source of true, lasting happiness could be found. It was the beginning of my studying the spiritual traditions of the East: Daoism, Zen, Hinduism, Tibetan Buddhism, and Sufism. And here I was now, twenty-five years later, the apprentice to a world famous Chinese Tonic Herbalist, whose clients were some of the most famous people on the planet but who weren't any happier than the people who buy tickets to their movies or listen to their music. This rekindled my longing to discover the source of true happiness that I knew dwelled within each of us as our True Nature.

When there was a break in the flow of clients that afternoon, Ron gave me a personal consultation. He took me into his consultation room, had me sit in a chair, and placed his fingers on the inner side of my wrists, thereby taking my pulses. Then he asked me to stick out my tongue. Two of the most important diagnostic tools in Chinese medicine, as well as Ayurvedic medicine and Siddha medicine, are pulse and tongue diagnosis. Through these diagnostic techniques, a skilled practitioner can obtain profound insight into a patient's condition on many levels, including the strength or weakness of all the major organs. Ron explained that his herbal teacher could even diagnose a person's Yin/Yang balance by listening to how their footsteps sounded as they walked down the hall and how they opened and closed the door to the consultation room. Ron then said that he was going to start me on my own tonic herbal program. He led me into the living room, took four bottles of capsules off the shelf, and handed them to me. They were Super Adaptogen, Supreme Protector, Imperial Garden, and Young at Heart.

These bottles contained capsules of spray-dried powders made from many of the most powerful and beneficial Chinese Tonic Herbs. Ron recommended that I take three capsules of each, twice a day. He emphasized that the first rule of Chinese Tonic Herbalism is compliance and said that if I took the herbs regularly I could notice benefits within months, or even weeks. At that point, I was around fifty years old and was beginning to feel the aging process starting to kick in. Although I had been a top athlete in school, since graduating I'd become sedentary, and lately I'd been sitting too many hours a day in front of a computer. Recently, I had begun to feel sluggish and was starting to feel aches and pains that I'd never noticed before. In the beginning of my apprenticeship, I would lumber up the stairs to Ron's office. After taking the herbs for three months I felt years younger, and after a year I felt ten years younger.

Soon I was bounding up the stairs and was enjoying an increase of energy, along with greater flexibility. My own personal experience of the benefits of Chinese Tonic Herbs was beginning.

Sometime during that first day, Ron brought me a book called *Rooted in Spirit: The Heart of Chinese Medicine* and handed it to me, saying, "This is the basis of Chinese Tonic Herbalism. Read it and you will have the foundation." I took the book to my room and read the back cover. It said:

"*Rooted in Spirit* explains the influence of the emotions on health according to ancient Chinese thought, examining the interrelationship of emotion and spirit and showing how our health and well-being depend upon the harmonious dwelling of the 'spirits' (shen) in the heart."

That night before going to sleep, I opened the book at random to page 64. I thought it was interesting that it was page 64 because when I was in high school I began studying the I-Ching, and there are 64 hexagrams in the I-Ching. On page 64 it said:

> *Thus, Knowing-How is the maintenance of life.*
> *Do not fail to observe the Four Seasons*
> *And to adapt to heat and cold,*
> *To Harmonize elation and anger,*
> *And to be calm in activity as in rest,*
> *To regulate the yin/yang,*
> *And to balance the hard and soft.*
>
> *In this way, having deflected the perverse energies,*
> *There will be long life and everlasting vision.*

Reading these words was the perfect end to my first day as Ron Teeguarden's apprentice. I felt that they contained wise instructions on how to succeed as his student as well as how to maintain my own health and master my life. I fell asleep feeling a deep sense of peace, happy to be where life had brought me, and inspired about what lay ahead.

3. HOW RON TEEGUARDEN DISCOVERED TONIC HERBS

As I settled into life in the herbarium, I got to know Ron better. We were born only one year apart, were roughly the same height, and people often thought that we were brothers. His kindness to me was like that of a big brother, and I came to consider him like the brother I never had. Naturally, I was curious how he had first learned about the Tonic Herbs. One day, he told me his personal story.

Ron attended the University of Michigan in Ann Arbor, as a pre-med student on an athletic scholarship (tennis). During his time in Ann Arbor, he started a natural foods co-op below a Maoist bookstore. It was the sixties, a time of much creativity and exploration. Eventually, Ron contracted a viral infection and lost 50 pounds. He suffered from extreme exhaustion, depression, and headaches and was so depleted of energy that he couldn't even walk to his job. All the doctors that he went to had no idea what was wrong or how to cure him.

One day, a friend who had gone to Toronto gave Ron a bottle of a Chinese herbal product that he had brought back from his trip. The formula was based on the herb He Shou Wu, or Polygonum which is known for its power of rejuvenation.

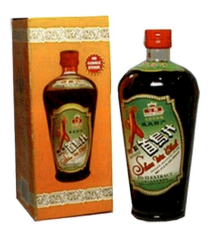

Ron's friend suggested that he try this herbal product, and he did. After all, he had nothing to lose. Not realizing that it was a concentrate meant to last a month, Ron drank the whole bottle in one day. The next day, to his amazement, he felt a lot better and bought a few more bottles. Within a week, the color had returned to his face, and he had regained his energy. So, a mistake had proven to him the effectiveness of the Chinese herbs. That marked the beginning of his belief in the healing power of the Chinese Tonic Herbs.

Now, having experienced first hand the benefits of Chinese herbs, Ron wanted to learn more. He heard about a Chinese man who lived in the San Fernando Valley of California, so Ron hitch-hiked across America and arrived on the man's doorstep, asking to be his student. When the man's wife answered the door, she didn't look happy to see a long-haired young stranger. The Chinese man took Ron to the backyard, which was barren, hard-packed earth. He handed Ron a shovel and told him to dig it up to make a garden. In true Karate Kid-style, Ron began his apprenticeship under the Asian teacher. Eventually, Ron returned to his home town of Los Angeles and opened a sports acupressure clinic in Santa Monica.

At this point, Ron had no idea what was about to happen that would radically transform his life. Soon he would meet his Daoist Herbal Master and would step onto the path that would lead him to become one of the pioneers of the health movement in America.

4. TONIC HERBALISM TAKES ROOT IN AMERICA

From the beginning of my apprenticeship under Master Herbalist Ron Teeguarden, my primary interest was how the Tonic Herbs had been used by the Daoist and Buddhist sages to promote spiritual development. I was overjoyed to be living in the home of a Daoist Herbal Master, and I took advantage of every opportunity to glean some understanding of the spiritual tradition associated with the Tonic Herbs.

My training was not conventional. There were no classes, but it was totally traditional, in the sense that I lived with the Master Herbalist and his family. The lessons were gained from everyday experience, rather than from textbooks. Much of the time, Ron was upstairs in his office, deeply involved in researching herbs or writing the most recent book that he was working on. I tried my best to avoid disturbing him, so as not to break his concentration. When a situation required that I interrupt him, Ron would take a short break in his writing to explain an important point about Tonic Herbalism. I cherished these profound downloads of herbal wisdom.

As I performed my daily duties of unpacking deliveries of herbs, keeping the drawers in the herbarium filled, and brewing custom teas, I constantly kept my ears open for the chance to overhear one of Ron Teeguarden's conversations with guests. Sometimes people who had known Ron for a long time would stop by for a consultation or simply to socialize. Some of these people were Ron's personal friends. Some were well-known yoga teachers and others were famous herbalists. These gatherings were a golden opportunity for me to take a break from my chores, serve them tea, and take a seat off to the side to absorb golden nuggets of herbal wisdom. I soaked up Ron's stories and seemed to have an innate capacity for remembering them. One day, one of the other employees at the herbarium said to me, "I don't know how you remember every one of Ron's stories, word for word. I can't remember even one." It's been scientifically proven that we learn and remember more from stories than from memorizing facts.

It was these stories that conveyed to me the essence of Chinese Tonic Herbalism.

My favorite stories were the ones about Ron's teacher, the Korean Daoist Herbalist Grand Master Sung Jin Park and his teacher, Moo San Do Sha, a Daoist Master in his 90s, who lived in the mountains of South Korea. The story goes that Master Park's teacher would meditate for three hours every morning, and the last hour was spent meditating under a waterfall. Moo San Do Sha spent his days walking the trails through the mountains, collecting wild Tonic Herbs. One day Master Park and Moo San Do Sha came upon a valley that had particularly good feng shui. Moo San Do Sha told Master Park that this spot had exceptionally powerful healing energy and that they should build a temple there, so that people would go there and benefit from the natural healing energy. The only problem was that they had no money to build a temple. So, Moo San Do Sha suggested that Master Park go to America and teach classes in Tonic Herbalism. That way he would spread the knowledge of Tonic Herbalism in the West, and then Master Park could return to Korea with the money he had been paid for the classes so that they could build the temple.

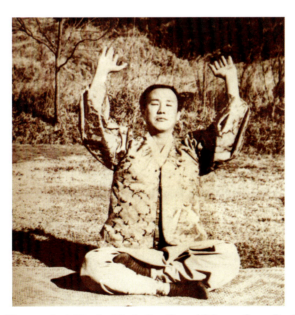

Ron Teeguarden's Daoist Herbalist Grand Master Sung Jin Park

That was how Master Park came to Los Angeles. It sounded good in theory, but at that time in Los Angeles, hardly anyone was interested in learning about Tonic Herbalism, so Master Park had to resort to teaching martial arts. Not only was he a great Tonic Herbalist, but he was also a black belt in several styles of martial arts and one of South Korea's top martial artists. Things weren't going so well. He hadn't come to America to teach martial arts, and he hated living in Los Angeles. He had been living in the pristine mountains of Korea with his Daoist sage master, bathing in waterfalls, and living on fresh wild Tonic Herbs. Now, he was living in a congested, polluted, and very materialistic city, where hardly anyone appreciated the profound wisdom that he had traveled so far to offer. Master Park tried over and over to give workshops, but no one came. Finally, exasperated to the point of wanting to give up and return to Korea, Master Park decided to try one last time to hold a workshop. He took out an advertisement in one of the free newspapers that they give away in Korea Town. That turned out to be a wise and fateful decision.

One day, in 1974, Ron happened to be in Korea Town and picked up one of those free newspapers. It was the only time in his life that he had looked at one of them, and noticing Master Park's advertisement, he decided to attend the workshop. When Ron arrived at the venue, there was only one other person there. Master Park came into the room, told them both to stand on their head against the wall, and then left. After standing on his head for over ten minutes, the other fellow came down off the wall and said, "This is crazy," and stormed out. When Master Park returned, he saw Ron still standing on his head and said, "Good. You are my student."

Ron instantly recognized the depth of Master Park's wisdom. Master Park began transmitting to Ron the inner principles of Tonic Herbalism that are very difficult to obtain even today without the direct guidance of a true Daoist Master Herbalist. Ron was teaching acupressure classes in Santa Monica at the time, and he soon began organizing classes in Tonic Herbalism for Master Park. Still to this day, in our travels we meet people who attended those early classes. Ron became Master Park's primary student. Eventually Master Park explained to Ron that he had promised his teacher,

Moo San Do Sha, that he would find ten students in America who would pass the knowledge of Tonic Herbalism on to ten more students. Master Park had only found Ron, and he asked Ron to make the same promise that he had made to his teacher, so that he could return to Korea. Ron gladly accepted this sacred honor and vowed to devote his life to spreading Tonic Herbalism in America and throughout the world.

This is how Ron Teeguarden eventually came to be recognized as the person who introduced Tonic Herbalism to America. I feel deeply honored to have been offered the opportunity to be his apprentice, to live with his family, and to receive from him the ancient wisdom of the Daoist Tonic Herbal Masters.

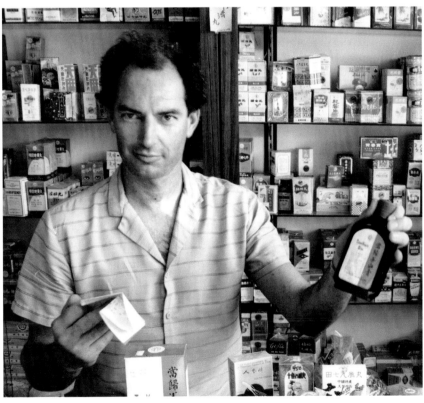

Ron Teeguarden in Los Angeles in the 1970s

5. THE THREE TREASURES PHILOSOPHY

Early in my apprenticeship with Daoist Herbal Master Ron Teeguarden, he began explaining to me the key to understanding Tonic Herbalism. It is called the Three Treasures Philosophy. It is an elegantly simple and yet ultimately profound understanding of how to develop the state of Radiant Health. In the years since I first learned of it, I have come to regard the Three Treasures Philosophy as China's greatest gift to the world.

As I write these words, it gives me great pleasure to share this knowledge with you, dear reader, because I know from personal experience the power of this system of health to radically improve one's quality of life and to make possible the attainment of enlightenment.

The ancient sages were students of Nature and of the human body. They were scientists who conducted research on the body, mind, and spirit in an attempt to maximize their functioning. The body was their laboratory, and their instrument of research was their attention. Over thousands of years, these sages devoted themselves to developing their consciousness in order to attain enlightenment. The attainment of the pinnacle of human consciousness requires not only a healthy body, for the body is the temple of the spirit, but also an alert and calm mind, free from the confusion of tumultuous thoughts. And finally, a peaceful spirit is required in order to reach the heights of spiritual attainment. The sages needed all three—body, mind, and spirit—to be in a state of harmony.

The sages of antiquity discovered that there were three basic energies in every human being. They called them Jing, Chi, and Shen.

Jing

Jing is our essential or primordial energy. It is hereditary. We get it from our parents. When the sperm of our father and the egg of our mother meet, their life-force produces our life-force. This energy, called Jing, is of tremendous importance to our health. Have you ever noticed how some people have weak constitutions and get sick frequently and others are extremely robust and rarely get sick? We inherit this Jing from our parents, and it is vitally important. When our Jing is strong, we are healthy, and when our Jing is totally depleted, our health fails. We age and die.

Our lifestyle strongly affects our Jing. If we burn the candle at both ends, don't eat well, don't get enough sleep, consume too much alcohol, cigarettes, or drugs, have too much sex, or work too hard, we deplete our Jing. This is what is often referred to as "burning out." When our Chi or daily energy runs out, we draw from our reserve of energy, our Jing, and when that tank runs dry, we die. Such is the case of those who die early deaths, like the "rock star lifestyle," characterized by overindulgence and a lack of moderation. Jing is consumed over our lifetime, and much of what people regard as the aging process is the result of the depletion of Jing.

The ancient sages discovered that there are certain herbs that can restore one's Jing. These Jing Tonics are the secrets of longevity. Longevity was important to the sages who were striving for enlightenment, because time was needed for the cultivation of spirit. The longer one lived, the more time could be spent on spiritual development. I have heard people say, "I don't want to have a very long life, because then I'll just be old and sick." It is entirely possible, through the regular use of the Tonic Herbs and by leading a balanced life of moderation, to remain extremely healthy, well beyond the years that most people today consider normal. Throughout history, there have been remarkable cases of great herbalist sages who lived healthy vital lives well past a hundred years, and some even older.

Chi

Chi can be thought of as our everyday energy. It is the energy that we are most familiar with because we depend upon it every day. When we wake up in the morning after a good night's sleep, we have plenty of energy and then, after consuming it all day long, we are tired at night. We are very aware of when we have a lot of Chi, and we are also very aware when we lack it. Our Chi is replenished by the food we eat, the water we drink, the air we breathe, and the sleep we get at night. The ancient herbalists discovered that there were certain herbs that nourished our Chi. These herbs are called Chi Tonics. In our modern lives, where our food is often nutritionally deficient, the water we drink is not pure, and the air is polluted, these Chi Tonics can be of great help by increasing our daily energy.

Shen

Finally, the ancient herbalist sages discovered Shen, or Spirit Tonics. Because these sages were striving for enlightenment, the cultivation of spirit was of tremendous importance to them. They strove to develop a calm spirit that was in harmony with the Dao, the flow of life. They discovered that there were herbs that promoted a calm spirit and that these herbs, when used in combination with meditation, elevated their awareness.

The ancient herbalists discovered that not only are there herbs that nourish specific treasures, but that some herbs, like Reishi and Schizandra, nourish all Three Treasures, making them the supreme Supertonic Herbs. This is why we try to consume Reishi and Schizandra every day of our life.

In *The Jade Emperor's Mind Seal Classic: A Taoist Guide to Health, Longevity, and Immortality*, translation and commentary by Stuart Alve Olson, it says:

> *"The supreme medicine" (shang yao), literally translates as "the foremost healing herbs." The full meaning of this medicine includes not only the idea of a preventative or curative prescription for physical illnesses, but also the idea of a "wonder drug" for all mental and spiritual illnesses. These "supreme medicines" are not something external to the self, but rather the very forces that constitute your existence. These forces are considered by the Taoist as three primary functions within each human being: jing, chi, and shen.*
>
> *The three energies are normally referred to in Taoist works*

as "The Three Treasures" (san bao). It is the preservation and cultivation of these three that promotes health, longevity, and immortality. Without these forces there can be no life, as it is their integration which constitutes existence. The degree of their abundance determines the level and quality of your health and the length of your life. Their transformation into "the elixir" brings about immortality.

When I first began to learn about "The Three Treasures" from my Daoist Herbalist Master Ron Teeguarden, so much about life began to make sense. The dots began to line up, and I saw clearly why so many people suffer from physical, mental, emotional, and spiritual dis-ease. I understood that the underlying causes of so much illness in our society was due to the lack of understanding of the importance of the Three Treasures. The majority of people engage in lifestyles that drain them of Chi and deplete their Jing, with no awareness of how to nurture Shen. Then, when they become unbalanced and develop symptoms of disease, they run to doctors, looking for a quick fix through drugs, many of which have negative side effects.

The good news is that Daoist Tonic Herbalists throughout the ages discovered and passed down to us knowledge of safe natural substances from the plant kingdom that replenish the Three Treasures so that we can live healthy, productive, and fulfilled lives. This is why I consider the Three Treasures Philosophy to be China's greatest gift to the world.

The great Chinese Daoist sage, Lu Zi, expressed this beautifully:

"The human body is only Jing, Qi, and Shen. These are the three treasures. These three treasures are complete as a human being. In order to attain true health and happiness, you must value the three treasures. Without the three treasures you cannot live long, and deep attainment cannot be reached in a lifetime. The three treasures must not be wasted. They must be nourished and protected as one's life."

6. THE HISTORY OF CHINESE HERBALISM

The origin of Tonic Herbalism and what is today known as Traditional Chinese Medicine (TCM) is lost in prehistory. The invention of writing occurred in the Shang Dynasty, that ruled China for around 400 years, from 1500 BCE to 1100 BCE. In the earliest Chinese writings, there are mentions of medicine being practiced in the pre-historic period. Herbs had already been used for several thousand years, so it is likely that these early healers were shamans who utilized herbs in their cures.

The first traditionally recognized herbalist in China is Shennong, who is said to have lived around 2800 BCE. Shennong has become a god-like mythical figure in China and is often depicted as a recluse wearing leaves. His name literally means "Divine Farmer" because he is regarded as the originator of agriculture in China. Before Shennong, it is believed that Chinese people ate mainly meat and wild fruits. It is said that he introduced a diet based on grains and vegetables. Shennong is believed to have lived nearly 5,000 years ago. This is why Chinese medicine is often said to be 5,000 years old.

Shennong is reported to have traveled throughout China and to have tasted every available herb. His *Shénnóng Běn Cao Jīng (Shennong's Materia Medica)* is considered to be the oldest book on Chinese herbal medicine. The original text of Shennong's *Materia Medica* has been lost, but there are extant translations. This book is of tremendous importance in the history of herbalism because in it Shennong classified 365 species of roots, grass, woods, furs, animals, and stones into three categories of herbal medicine. These three categories are:

1. Substances that must be taken in small doses as treatments for specific illnesses. These are what we call today the "medicinal herbs." These herbs are effective, but must be taken only for a prescribed period of time.

2. Tonics that must also not be taken for long periods of time.

3. The final category is the "Superior Herbs." These are the Tonic Herbs that can restore balance in the body and maintain a state of Radiant Health. These herbs have no negative side effects, so they can be consumed every day of one's life. In fact, in China people throughout the ages have cooked with these herbs every day to promote health and well being.

There is an important lesson that we can learn from Shennong's approach to herbalism. Today many students of TCM, during their training, study the names and properties of various herbs that they learn about from books. However, they have little hands-on experience, tasting each herb and substance like Shennong did. This personal experience with the herbs is highly informative and beneficial—in fact, you could say that it is essential for becoming a Master Herbalist.

During the generations that followed, many succeeding herbalists added to the herbal knowledge that Shennong had recorded for posterity. Probably the most significant of these latter works is Li Shizhen's *Compendium of Materia Medica (Bencao Gangmu)* that was written in the Ming dynasty. This text is still used today by practicing herbalists in China and throughout the world. Li Shizhen (1518–1593) is by far the most highly respected herbalist and medical scholar in the history of China. His portrait is displayed in virtually every traditional medical school in China. Li Shizhen is famous throughout China and is highly respected, not only by herbalists. To give you an idea of how highly Li Shizhen is respected in China, the world famous martial arts actor Jet Li once said that Li Shizhen is the person that he most looks up to.

Li Shizhen spent nearly forty years traveling all over China. He studied all the available books on herbs, researched folk remedies, and personally experienced the effects of a vast number of herbs. He interviewed many herbal doctors, including his own father and grandfather. One of the reasons that he was so dedicated in his pursuit of herbal knowledge was that he felt that many of the existing herbal texts had inaccurate information that could be harmful to patients. So, he attempted to compile accurate and verifiable information that could be of lasting benefit to people.

Unfortunately, his text was so detailed that it was too large for traveling doctors to carry with them on their rounds, and it had to be divided into several books. Li Shizhen wanted the court to publish his master work, but they stored it away. Finally, in 1644, an edition with high quality illustrations of herbs was published. Today, it is widely regarded to be the greatest scientific achievement of the Ming era. It is largely due to the efforts of Li Shizhen that China developed what is considered by many to be the most highly respected herbal system in the world.

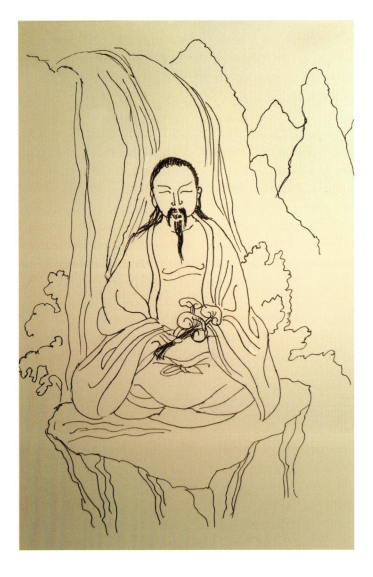

7. DAOIST MOUNTAIN HERMITS— LIVING IN HARMONY WITH NATURE

Since my main focus in life was spiritual development and attaining enlightenment, I was particularly interested in the Daoist and Buddhist sages who had practiced Tonic Herbalism. Some of the herbalists who developed Chinese herbalism throughout the ages had served in the courts of Chinese royalty as Master Herbalists. They were responsible for researching and recording the efficacy of herbal formulas in the improvement of health and attainment of longevity. There was another class of great herbalists who lived in monasteries and developed herbal cures for the benefit of the monks and lay people. But yet another category of Master Herbalists lived outside of royal courts and monasteries. They were the Daoist and Buddhist hermits, yogis, and recluses who lived quiet lives in Nature. The Daoist path advocated simplicity, living one's life in harmony with the Dao, according to the Laws of Nature. This was the group of Master Herbalists that interested me the most.

Throughout Chinese literature, one reads about sages of ancient times that are revered because they lived extremely long lives according to the Dao. Ever since childhood, I intuitively felt that our western materialistic society was out of harmony with Nature. My happiest times in childhood were spent running through the woods and jumping over streams. As I grew older, it pained me to see our disconnect with Nature. Like Joni Mitchell sang, "They paved paradise and put up a parking lot." When I met Ron Teeguarden and was invited to move into his house as his apprentice, I felt that a door had opened that would allow me to reconnect with the beauty and power of Nature, and I knew that this was essential in order to attain enlightenment.

The ancient wisdom of Tonic Herbalism was passed down through the ages by the lineage of Daoist and Buddhist Herbal Masters, many of whom were hermits living in the mountains of China and Korea. Like Ron Teeguarden's Daoist teacher, Grand Master Sung Jin Park, and his teacher, Moo San Do Sha, who lived in the mountains of South Korea, these monks preferred to live far away from the din of society and enjoyed the solitude of Nature. Theirs was not just an avoidance of the ordinary concerns of society but was rather an intentional movement to harmonize with Nature. Their lifestyle of living high in remote mountains and consuming wild Tonic Herbs allowed them to plumb the depths of Nature, meditate deeply, and become one with the flow of Nature's movements. The effects of the herbs that they consumed daily were well known, for they had been studied by their teachers, and their teacher's teachers, for literally millennia. These masters knew from their own experience that some herbs increased Chi, thereby giving one more energy. Some herbs restored one's primal energy, Jing, and thereby promoted longevity. And some herbs nourished Shen (Spirit), calming the mind and promoting a feeling of being more centered, thereby enhancing meditation and spiritual development. Furthermore, these mountain hermits held several herbs like Reishi Mushroom and Schizandra in extreme reverence because these herbs nourished all Three Treasures: Jing, Chi, and Shen.

Most of us cannot or do not want to live the same lifestyle as these mountain hermits. Our modern world is largely cut off from Nature. Many people who live in urban areas are surrounded by glass and concrete buildings all day and rarely get to enjoy even an hour sitting under a tree and watching the clouds float by, let alone bathing in a mountain stream or eating wild herbs. Being so disconnected from Nature, it stands to reason that modern people often feel a malaise, an inner feeling that something just isn't right. This inner discontent manifests in depression and anxiety, two of the plagues so prevalent in modern life. The use and abuse of anti-anxiety and anti-depression drugs is skyrocketing, but there is another solution. Perhaps we should take advantage of what our ancestors learned about the plants that can restore our harmony with Nature. There is a tendency in the modern world to think we have all the answers and that science can solve anything. But, what good are the latest technological gadgets if we lack health of body and peace of mind and spirit? The Tonic Herbs can be utilized, while living in the modern world, to bring us back into balance, and maybe once that balance has been restored, we will also see how to adjust our personal lifestyle to become more healthy, happy, and fulfilled.

8. DAOIST LONGEVITY TECHNIQUES

Throughout the ages, Daoists placed great emphasis on health and longevity. In their pursuit of longevity, Daoists have utilized three main techniques:

- the use of herbal formulas
- physical and breathing exercises to move the Chi within certain energetic channels
- meditation to promote tranquility of heart, mind, and body

Even practicing just one of these three techniques in a dedicated manner will greatly enhance one's health and longevity. However, for people who are serious about attaining heights of spiritual development, they would be well advised to practice all three: herbs, physical and breathing exercises, along with meditation. If all three are practiced regularly, it is entirely possible that one could enjoy good health for over 100 years.

Western society overly celebrates youth. When you travel to Asian countries, you find that they have much more respect for the elderly. Elderly people are not disrespected and discarded like they are in the West but are valued for their wisdom.

Many Daoist teachers have lived over 100 years. In Daoist circles, enjoying youthfulness for a life-span of 100 years has long been considered to be proof of the veracity of one's teachings. For Daoists who were interested in self-cultivation, it was important to remain youthful for a long time. Self-cultivation takes time, and if one is unhealthy then one would not have the required energy to persevere in their practice. And if one died at a young age, then obviously self-cultivation would come to a premature end before one succeeded in attaining the goal.

There is an ancient tradition in China of associating certain mountains with particular Daoist and Buddhist sages who dwelled deep in the mountains and lived entirely on wild herbs. These sacred mountains are highly revered in China and are places of pilgrimage where hundreds of thousands of Chinese visit each year. It is believed that many of those sages attained "immortality" and that their enlightened energy can still be felt on those sacred summits.

In Chinese, the word "immortality" means "man of the mountains." Many of these mountain men were hermits who were striving to become one with Nature—one with the Dao. Ron Teeguarden's Daoist Master, Sung Jin Park, and his master, Moo San Do Sha, were such men of the mountains. They wandered throughout the mountains of Korea gathering Tonic Herbs that were their exclusive diet. They also practiced physical and breathing exercises, which is evidenced by the fact that Master Park was one of Korea's top martial artists, having black belts in several martial arts. In addition, Master Park told Ron that his teacher used to meditate every morning for three hours and would spend the last hour under a waterfall. Obviously, Master Moo San Do Sha was an advanced meditator.

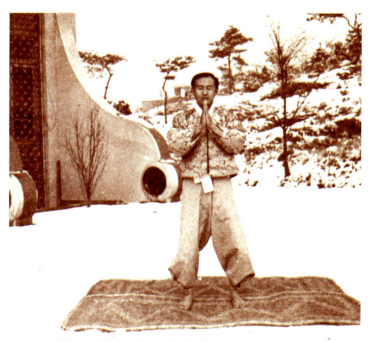

Daoist Master Sung Jin Park practicing Qigong

Central to the pursuit of longevity was the preservation and maintenance of the Three Treasures: Jing, Chi, and Shen. Ingesting Tonic Herbs was fundamental to this process of self-cultivation. Herbs that increased one's Jing boosted one's vitality. Herbs that increased one's Chi energized one's activity. Herbs that increased one's Shen nourished one's Spirit.

Next, the practice of Qigong contributed to mastering the accumulation and movement of Chi in the body. Daoist and Buddhist monks, who practiced self-cultivation, became aware in meditation of energy (Chi) moving along certain channels to specific areas of their body. Over thousands of years, these energy channels were recorded and a highly sophisticated system developed that described the flow of energy in the body. The understanding of energy meridians that acupuncture is based upon is one of China's greatest contributions to the world. The Tonic Herbs tonify vital organs through specific meridians. Master Park told Ron that Schizandra was his favorite Tonic Herb because it tonifies all Three Treasures, enters all twelve meridians, and nurtures all five elements.

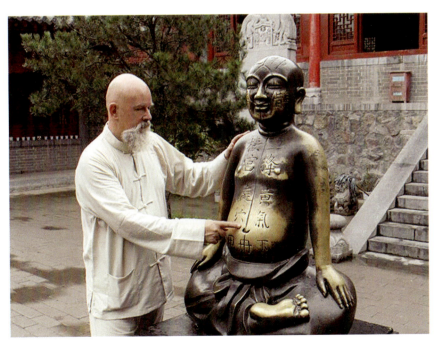

Ganga inspecting a statue at the Shaolin Temple showing meridians

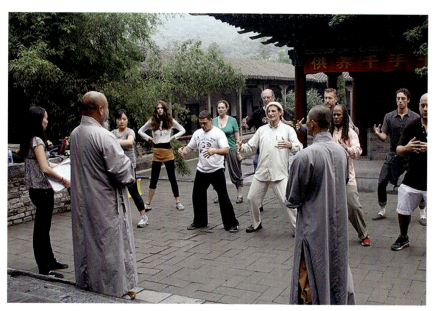
Receiving a Qigong class from senior monks at the Shaolin Temple

Qigong is a highly complex and detailed system that includes many techniques. However, there is one practice that is considered to be the oldest and the foundation of all other Qigong techniques. It is called the Eight Silken Brocades (Baduanjin). The Eight Silken Brocades gets its name from its smooth flowing movements and is primarily practiced as a form of medical Qigong in order to improve health. The series of eight simple exercises has been practiced in China for over 1,000 years. Because of its age, many styles of the Eight Silken Brocades have developed over time. Different monasteries, like Shaolin and Wudang, developed their own unique styles of the Eight Silken Brocades, and also certain teachers developed their own styles. There may be slight differences in style, but the exercises are essentially the same.

Anyone interested in practicing the Daoist Longevity Techniques is recommended to learn and practice the Eight Silken Brocades. When we visited the Shaolin Temple with Ron and his wife, we received a class in the Eight Silken Brocades from advanced monks.

It was an experience that I will never forget. But, if you can't travel to China to visit the Shaolin Temple, there are easily over 50 videos on YouTube that you can watch for free. Watch several until you find one that appeals to you and then practice it regularly. A requirement in Qigong practice is to maintain relaxation and deep breathing that facilitates the flow of Chi. Each exercise improves the health of specific internal organs and the entire series of Eight Silken Brocades can be completed in around fifteen minutes.

Regular daily practice of the Eight Silken Brocades, combined with the regular use of Chinese Tonic Herbs, plus meditation, will transform your life. These are the techniques that the great sages of China and Korea practiced with great success. These three modalities, when combined, improve the functioning of internal organs, increase vitality, develop greater clarity of mind, and ultimately result in higher states of consciousness, culminating in enlightenment, becoming a man or woman who is one with the Dao.

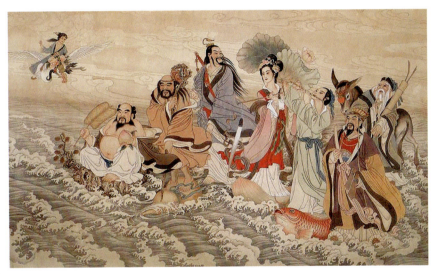

Eight Daoist Immortals

Jing Qi Shen Xuan Guan

This Chinese phrase can be translated as
"The Three Treasures are the Entrance
to the State of Conscious Immortality."

9. THE BEST OF THE ANCIENT AND MODERN

We are living in a very exciting time. We have available to us today an abundance of high quality Tonic Herbs. Mainly due to modern transportation systems and increased trade between distant countries, we have access to herbs like Rhodiola that grows at the snowline in Tibet, Cordyceps from Bhutan, Wild Reishi from Changbai Mountain, and Snow Lotus from the Himalayas. Never before in the history of the world has it been possible to so easily obtain such a variety of high quality herbs.

In ancient times, these precious herbs were harvested in remote places that few people had access to. Then, the herbs were transported by caravan via routes like the Silk Road to the capital of China. It is said that if you were granted an audience with the Empress of China, the present that she prized most highly was Snow Lotus that grows high in the Himalayas. This rare herb actually blossoms in the snow and is famous as a beauty tonic, due to improving the health of the skin and developing a radiant complexion.

Today we are doubly blessed, because we also have at our disposal the most scientifically advanced technologies for the production of tonic herbal supplements. We are indebted to the lineage of ancient tonic herbalists who passed down this profound knowledge to us, and we are also fortunate to be able use the latest advanced technology to extract the essence of these herbs for our benefit.

Ron Teeguarden uses the most modern, scientifically advanced, manufacturing techniques. All of his Dragon Herbs products are produced in state-of-the art herbal manufacturing facilities.

In 1993, Ron was on a flight to Beijing and just happened to be sitting next to Xiao Pei-Gen, who was the Commissioner of Drug Approval for the People's Republic of China. You can imagine how surprised Professor Xiao was when Ron opened his carry-on bag and showed him that he was traveling with an article written by Professor Xiao called "The Anti-Aging Herbs of China." Professor Xiao has been called "a living pharmacopoeia of TCM" and has published more than 500 scientific papers and twenty scientific books. This was a highly auspicious meeting because after this long plane flight Professor Xiao became Ron's main mentor in China. Their friendship allowed Ron to have access to the most advanced herbal institute in China, Professor Xiao's world famous Institute of Materia Plant Development. This led to Ron having access to China's top scientists, herbal research institutions, and manufacturing facilities. But equally important was the fact that Ron now had access to sources of the highest quality herbs in China.

An excellent example of how Ron Teeguarden's Dragon Herbs is at the leading edge of herbal manufacturing is FITT™, Fingerprint Identical Transfer Technology™. This is a proprietary extraction technology that captures the original phyto-chemical profile of a plant and transfers it safely and almost identically into the final extraction. Not only is the plant's "fingerprint" transferred, but in addition the aroma, color, and taste of the plant are perfectly preserved. The entire manufacturing process is controlled under 104° F, so FITT™ is considered to be a raw extraction.

This is one example of why Ron Teeguarden's Dragon Herbs are widely regarded to be the highest quality Tonic Herbs available in the world.

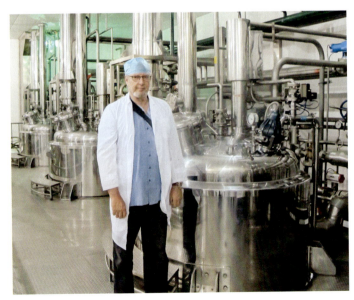

Ron Teeguarden in a state-of-the-art herbal factory

10. BECOMING A TEA MASTER

After working for Dragon Herbs for a year, I was given the title of Tea Master. My duties were two-fold. When clients arrived at the house, I would greet them at the front door and show them into the living room. As they entered the living room, they passed by a large wood counter that had been carved from a tree trunk. I stood behind this counter next to a three-foot-tall brass urn, where I would offer to make them a tonic elixir. I used what's called a siphon, that looks kind of like something you'd find in a chemistry lab. Ron had discovered these siphons being used to make coffee at hotels in China and had realized their usefulness in making tonic elixirs. On the countertop I had a full assortment of wonderful herbal tonic tinctures that I could add, according to what the client needed.

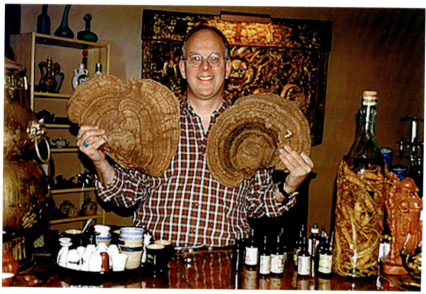

Ganga behind the Elixir Bar with giant Reishi Mushrooms

The procedure was simple and a lot of fun for the clients to watch. I'd place water in the spherical glass bowl on the bottom of the siphon, add raw herbs like Schizandra, Goji Berries, Asparagus Root, and Albizzia Flowers in the glass beaker on top, and then light the flame underneath. When the water boiled, it would flow up to the beaker on top and cook the herbs. At that point, I'd add a few squirts of tinctures, like 8 Immortals, Duanwood Reishi, and Supreme Shen Drops. After the concoction had boiled sufficiently, I would turn off the flame, and when the beaker on the bottom cooled, the vacuum would suck the brewed elixir down into the lower beaker. People enjoyed watching this process, and they really loved the elixirs. Quite often they would come in stressed, having driven through the heavy traffic that Los Angeles is known for, and after drinking a few of these tonic elixirs they would be feeling quite mellow and happy. I loved seeing the change that the tonics brought about in their mood and energy level. If they came in dragging their feet, the Chi Tonics increased their energy. And, if they came in down and depressed, the Shen Tonics had the wonderful effect of making them feel calm, as well as elevating their mood naturally. By my making these elixirs for the clients, it gave Ron a chance to focus on his writing upstairs in his office, and it gave the clients a chance to decompress from the hectic pace of living in Los Angeles.

My other main duty was cooking the custom teas. That task gave me the opportunity to handle all the Tonic Herbs on a daily basis. Actually touching and holding the raw herbs was a very important part of my training. You start to form a relationship with the herbs by handling them and knowing them energetically. I began to feel that each herb was a friend from the plant kingdom that had the power to restore people's health, balance their body, mind, and spirit, and promote Radiant Health.

When Ron did a consultation with a client, if they wanted a custom tea, he would write up a formula for them and pass it to me for brewing. We kept these formulas on file, and when it was time to prepare another batch of their custom tea, I would take that list of herbs and weigh out the prescribed amount of each herb. Then, I'd place the herbs in a canvas bag, and after cooking the herbs for about an hour, turn the valve to start the bagging process. When the boiling tea flowed into the bagging machine, aromatic steam would rise up and fill the room. It was so potent that you could smell the delightful aroma throughout the entire house.

I would fill sixty plastic pouches with the freshly brewed custom tea and then box up the pouches to be mailed to the client. Some days I had so many custom teas to prepare that I would work until 1 or 2 in the morning. I enjoyed the process because while the herbs were boiling for an hour, I could read a spiritual book. I was mainly reading books on Chinese Daoism and Chan (Zen) and would often dream of going to China one day. I would look at the picture that Ron had on his wall of Shennong, and I felt very fortunate that I had the opportunity to be the apprentice of a true Daoist Herbal Master.

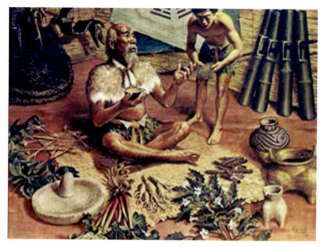

Master Herbalist Shennong and disciple

Late one night I was in the tea room when Ron poked his head in the door. He asked me how it was going and then asked if I had a passport. When I replied, "No," he said, "You'd better get one fast. We're going to China, and you're going with us." Ron told me that he and his wife, Yanlin, were going on an herbal expedition to Changbai Mountain, which is the source of many of the highest quality herbs in the world, and they wanted me to document the trip in video and still photos. I could hardly believe my ears. I had been wanting to go to China for over thirty years, and now my dream was about to come true.

In one year, since becoming Ron's apprentice, I had gone from knowing next to nothing about herbs to having the title of Tea Master. It had been a process of total immersion, living in the home of a Master Herbalist, being surrounded by the finest Tonic Herbs in the world, and brewing custom teas and elixirs every day. But most importantly, I had the opportunity to observe the changes that the Tonic Herbs brought about in people's lives.

One case that comes to mind was that of one of the most famous singers in the world. The day she first arrived for a consultation, she walked in slumped over, listless, and with dull eyes. She had just canceled her upcoming tour because she just didn't have the energy to go out on the road. She was given a Tonic Herbal program, and when she returned a month later, she walked in upright, with a spring in her step and a sparkle in her eyes. She finished the album she was working on, received critical acclaim, went out on the road, and had the most successful tour of her career.

It was these improvements that I observed in others, as well as myself, that convinced me of the amazing power of the Tonic Herbs to help people live productive and fulfilling lives. And now I was going to China, a dream come true, with a Master Daoist Tonic Herbalist to obtain the finest herbs in the world. Life was good. Very, very good.

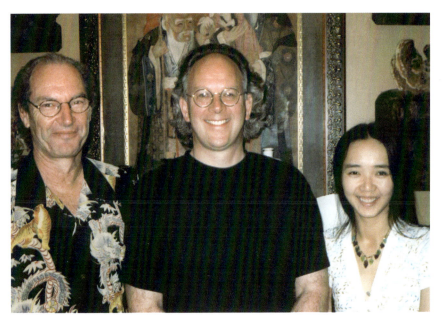

Ron and Yanlin Teeguarden with Ganga, the happy apprentice

11. THE FIRST NIGHT IN BEIJING— SEEING THE GOJI LADY

We were leaving for China in just a few weeks, so I rushed out the next day and applied for a passport and visa to China. As our departure date approached, my excitement increased and thoughts of ancient Buddhist and Daoist temples filled my mind. Finally, the day of our departure came and Ron, Yanlin, and I flew to Beijing. On the plane, I studied the manual for the new video camera that Ron had purchased, hoping that I wouldn't make any major mistakes using it. Twelve hours later, we landed in Beijing. As we took the taxi from the airport to the heart of Beijing, the roadside was lined with billboards advertising well-known multinational corporations. That was the first hint that my romantic idea of ancient China was no longer the modern day reality of the New China.

We checked in to a high-rise hotel on Wangfujing Street, which is the main commercial avenue of Beijing, the equivalent of Fifth Avenue in New York. I joined Ron and Yanlin for dinner in the hotel dining room, and afterwards Ron mentioned that he and Yanlin were tired from traveling and were going to go to bed early. When I said that I'd do the same, Ron exclaimed, "This is your first night in China. You should go out and see the town." I hesitatingly replied, "Well okay, I'll walk around, but I'll stay on the main roads." Ron said, "Oh, this is China. There's very little crime. You can walk anywhere you like." Emboldened by encouragement from my Daoist Herbal Master, I headed out into the night to experience my first night in China.

The first thing that I noticed was how clean everything was. The street was a beautifully landscaped pedestrian promenade, and the people were not dressed in drab Mao suits but rather looked like what you'd expect to see in New York, London, or Paris. I walked into the first shopping mall that I came to and was amazed at what I saw. It was the most elegant mall I'd ever seen. Now I understood what Ron and Yanlin had told me many months earlier, when Yanlin's parents were coming to visit. I had naively asked Yanlin,

"Are you going to take your parents to one of the best best shopping malls in Los Angeles?" thinking that they'd be impressed. Ron had said to me, "There isn't a shopping mall in America that would impress them." Now, I got it. China's economy was booming and the Chinese were leapfrogging over America. My impression of China was based on outdated media reports, but in the last thirty years China had become the world's fastest growing economy with growth rates approaching 10%.

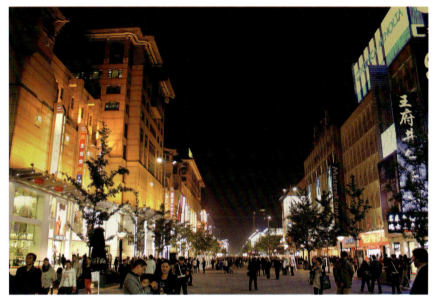

Wangfujing Street in Beijing

Starting in 1978, Deng Xiaoping broke with Mao's faulty economic policies by combining socialist ideology with more pragmatic market economic practices. He opened China to foreign investment and allowed private ownership in many sectors of the economy that had previously been state run. He is given credit for developing China into one of the fastest growing economies in the world. As I made my way down Wangfujing Street, I passed shopping mall after shopping mall, filled with luxury stores like Prada, Hermes, Armani, Dior, Gucci, Louis Vuitton, and Cartier. Evidently, the economic reforms introduced by Deng Xiaoping had created a lot of very wealthy Chinese.

But, shopping malls and luxury brands weren't what I was looking for. I was in search of the Old China, not the New China. So, I turned off the main street and headed down a side street, then turned onto a smaller street, and even a smaller street, then an alley, and found myself walking into a hutong. The hutongs were the traditional residential neighborhoods of China. They were a labyrinth of densely arranged one-story buildings, linked together by narrow alleyways. Families often washed their clothes and cooked in the narrow alleys. Due to the rapid modernization of China, the hutongs were quickly disappearing. It was not uncommon to find an entire city block, where just a few months earlier there had been historic hutongs, now bulldozed to make way for the construction of modern high-rise apartment buildings.

Somehow, despite it being dark and the fact that I was in a major Asian city for the first time, I made my way deeper and deeper into the hutong. It was like I was craving an experience of the old traditional China, far away from the glitz of luxury stores. The alleyways got narrower and narrower until they were only wide enough for one person to pass, and it was so dark that I could barely see. An old man suddenly appeared from the shadows and squeezed past me. Finally, I decided that maybe that was far enough and that if I was mugged, robbed, or killed, Ron and Yanlin would have no idea where I had disappeared to. So, I turned around and made my way back to the main street.

I felt a rush of adrenaline and was overwhelmed with the feeling that I was in the most exciting country I'd ever experienced. China was not only one of the world's most ancient cultures on Earth, that had invented the printing press, gunpowder, paper making, and the compass, but in a few decades it had become a major superpower. It was also home to three major religions: Daoism, Confucianism, and Buddhism, and this was where my interests lay. I felt a strong affinity with ancient China and knew that I'd spent many past lifetimes there.

As I walked toward the hotel, I wanted to squeeze just a little more experience out of my first night China. It was past midnight, but just a few blocks from the hotel I passed a tea shop that looked

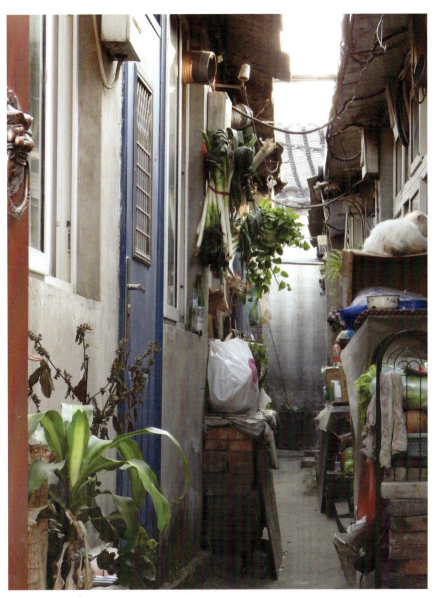

A Beijing hutong

open. It was the only store that I'd seen all night that looked traditional. I peered in the window and saw that despite the late hour, customers were still sitting around tables drinking tea. I entered, sat down, and felt instantly at home. Much of the decor was similar to Ron and Yanlin's home back in Los Angeles. A cheerful young waitress did her best attempting to wait on me. Even though she didn't speak more than a few words of English and I didn't speak any Chinese, I managed to order a pot of oolong tea. Holding a conversation was difficult, so we drew a lot of pictures. Before leaving, I managed to ask her if she would show me around Beijing the following day, and she agreed.

I walked back to the hotel feeling totally exhilarated after my first night in China. As I walked down the hotel hallway, I saw a middle-aged Chinese woman leave Ron and Yanlin's room. As she walked toward me, getting closer and closer, I noticed that she looked like the most healthy, vibrant woman I'd ever seen. She oozed vitality and radiated powerful, yet calm, clear energy. When she passed me, I nodded in greeting and then knocked on Ron and Yanlin's door. Ron opened the door and said, "You just missed the Goji Lady. She's the one who we buy our Goji Berries from. Her farm is at the base of Heaven Mountain." I told Ron that I had passed her in the hallway and had never seen a woman who looked that healthy. In America, we say, "An apple a day keeps the doctor away." In China, they believe that a handful of Goji Berries keeps you so healthy that you don't need doctors.

I fell asleep that night feeling that the immense world of Chinese culture had opened up for me to explore. I felt incredibly grateful to my Daoist Herbal Master Ron Teeguarden, and his wife Yanlin, for bringing me on this herbal expedition and looked forward to what amazing experiences lay ahead.

12. A CHINESE HERB MARKET

The next morning, we went on a day-trip to one of the largest herb markets in China. There are several of these, positioned in specific areas around China where regional herb farmers bring their produce. This market was a several-hour taxi ride outside of Beijing. When we arrived at the herb market, I was totally amazed. The market was inside a building that was the size of a major convention center in America, and it contained nothing but herbs of every kind.

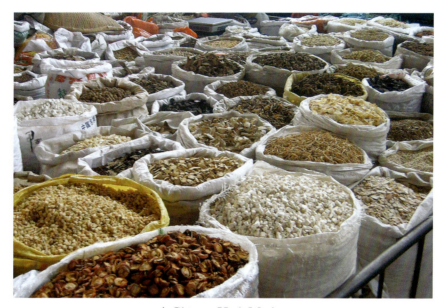

A Chinese Herb Market

One of the main reasons why Ron Teeguarden is recognized as a world famous Master Herbalist is that he never settles for less than the highest quality herbs. Once he has obtained that highest quality, he then continues looking for even higher quality.

Ron explained to me that a particular herb, for example Ginseng, might have ten grades, ranging from extremely poor quality all the way to the highest quality. Most herb companies purchase somewhere in the middle of that range to slightly higher, maybe from

5–7 on the scale. They can't buy the highest quality because they have to compete with other companies' products on the shelves in the stores. They have to meet a price point, and therefore settle on less than the absolute highest quality. But Ron's philosophy is based on ancient Daoist principles. He believes that "Health is All," and that nothing is more important than your health. You can be fabulously wealthy, but what good is it if you have poor health? The ancient Daoist herbalists throughout the ages have discovered how to utilize the Tonic Herbs to develop Radiant Health, and following in their tradition, Ron constantly searches for the finest of the fine. After all, if you're going to be spending money for your health, why not make sure that what you buy will really produce the benefits?

It was a wonderful experience for me to walk the aisles of the herb market, seeing firsthand where the herbs that reach America come from. Our next stop was a well-known herb shop where Ron wanted to see some very large and very old Ginseng roots. The better herb shops in China often have on display framed very old Ginseng roots hanging on the wall. You can tell the age of a Ginseng root by counting the nodules on its stem. Just like you can tell the age of a tree by counting the rings, you can also tell how old a Ginseng root is by how many nodules it has. Each nodule represents one year.

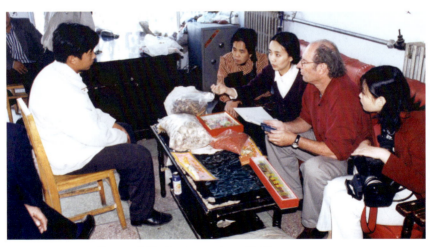

Ron and Yanlin inspecting old Ginseng roots

The owner of the shop brought out several large cases of Ginseng roots. Some were two or three feet long and could be hundreds of years old. Connoisseurs of Ginseng roots might purchase these to display in their home or store. I was quite impressed, but Ron reached into a bag, brought out a magnifying glass, and started closely examining the roots. After a thorough examination, he whispered to me, "They're fakes." When we got to the car, Ron explained to me that some dishonest merchants glue several roots together to make them appear older. They are so good at it that to your naked eye you would never know, but by examining with a magnifying glass, you can see where the roots are glued together. I was happy to have learned another practical lesson from my Daoist Herbal Master.

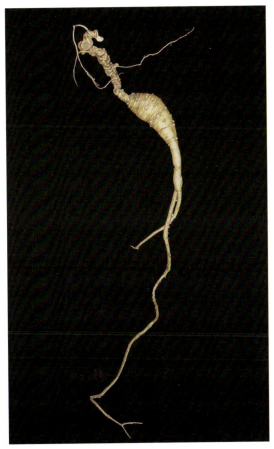

Genuine very old Ginseng root (notice the nodules at top)

13. DI DAO

One day, Ron introduced to me a wonderful Chinese concept known as Di Dao that literally means "Earth Dao" or "the Way of the Earth."

Note: Throughout this book, I have been using "Dao" rather than "Tao." "Dao" is the modern "pinyin" way to spell "Tao."

Ron explained that a Di Dao herb comes from the place that is traditionally associated with that herb. In other words, it means that the herb is genuine, authentic, and not from an inferior or counterfeit source. That is why we were on our way to Changbai Mountain in search of the highest quality Reishi and Ginseng. We could have easily gone to a major herb market near Beijing, where distributors market herbs that come from farms located throughout China. While that would have been much easier than trekking all the way to Changbai Mountain in northeast China on the border of Jilin Province and North Korea, it would not satisfy Ron's dedication to only provide to his customers the highest quality herbs. Changbai Mountain is famous in China because it is where the Emperor's Ginseng Gardens were located. It is well known by Master Herbalists that Changbai Mountain is the source of the highest quality herbs that are growing in a pristine environment with soil that is rich in minerals.

All plants that are growing anywhere in the world are influenced by their environmental conditions, such as temperature, rainfall, soil, humidity, and air quality. In addition, farmers in different areas may practice varying systems of agriculture that also influence the plant. How the plants are grown, harvested, and processed also have impact on the final product. Hence, the Chinese herbal industry places huge emphasis on Di Dao. In fact, the Chinese Pharmacopoeia states that all herbal products manufactured and sold in China must utilize Di Dao herbs in order to ensure that the herbs have come from a legitimate and genuine source. This is why Ron and his wife, Yanlin, travel extensively all over China in order to obtain Di Dao herbs directly from authentic sources.

Ron Teeguarden does not only obtain herbs exclusively from China. Many of the most famous Tonic Herbs come from China, but there are also wonderful Tonic Herbs that come from many other countries around the world. Ron obtains herbs from Tibet, Bhutan, Korea, Japan, Mongolia, Africa, New Zealand, Europe, Indonesia, Russia, and North and South America.

Another perfect example of how Ron sources Di Dao herbs is Heaven Mountain® Goji Berries that are sold by Dragon Herbs. I have eaten Goji Berries from stores all over China and America. All too often they are hard and dry, but Heaven Mountain Goji Berries® are soft, plump, and juicy. Heaven Mountain is a remote mountain range in the northern region of Xin Jiang Province, China. Ron obtains his Goji Berries from a farm that is at the base of Heaven Mountain. The water that irrigates this farm comes from the melted snow from glaciers on pristine Heaven Mountain. Everything about this environment—the water, soil, amount of sunshine, and weather conditions—is conducive to producing the best Goji Berries on Earth. Not only are they moist and juicy, but they are also extremely potent. Heaven Mountain Goji Berries are officially certified by China's Ministry of Agriculture as being Di Dao. This is how Ron makes sure that every herb that he provides through Dragon Herbs is the best available. You can say that Di Dao is the guiding principle by which Ron Teeguarden ensures the quality of Dragon Herbs and why his products are so highly respected around the world.

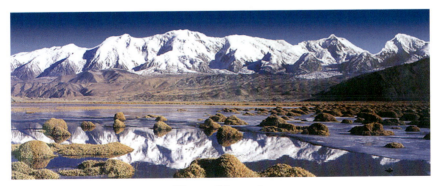

Heaven Mountain

14. EXPEDITION TO CHANGBAI MOUNTAIN

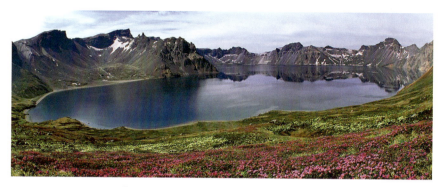

Heaven Lake at Changbai Mountain

The herbal expedition that I was fortunate to be on had a specific goal. Ron had heard that there was a Reishi Mushroom farm on Changbai Mountain that was growing the highest quality Reishi Mushrooms ever seen.

Changbai Mountain is famous for being the place where many of the highest quality herbs in the entire world grow. It is a dormant volcano with a lake at the top, called Heaven Lake, that is a lot like Crater Lake in Oregon. One of the reasons why the herbs that grow on the slopes of Changbai Mountain are so potent is that the soil there is very high in minerals. This is where the private Ginseng gardens of the Emperor of China were located.

When Ron first told me that he was taking me on an expedition to Changbai Mountain, I felt that it was more than just a trip to gather herbs. It was a pilgrimage to a sacred place. The very first day that I had met Ron, he had shown me a painting of the goddess Magu carrying a Reishi Mushroom. The Chinese believe that Magu brought the Reishi Mushroom down from Heaven to Changbai Mountain for humanity. Changbaishan, or Eternally White Mountain as it is known in Chinese, is the tallest peak in Northeast China and is considered one of the five holy mountains of Korea.

Naturally, when I heard that we were going to Changbai Mountain, I began to research the mountain on the internet. I discovered that the Changbaishan National Nature Reserve covers a total area of 2,000 square kilometers. It is a large natural flora and fauna Nature Reserve and a part of the UNESCO's Man and Biosphere Program. In addition to Heaven Lake, on its slopes are many waterfalls, hot springs, and pristine forests where many varieties of Tonic Herbs grow wild. The mountain has a very large selection of flora, consisting of 80 different types of trees and over 300 medicinal plant species. It is literally on the border of China and North Korea. Heaven Lake is 1,260 feet deep and 8 miles in circumference, but you cannot walk all the way around it because one side of it is in North Korea. The Erdaobai River runs off of Heaven Lake and creates the tallest volcanic waterfall in the world, which is 223 feet high.

This sacred natural wonderland was our destination. We flew from Beijing to the nearest city at the base of Changbai Mountain. The next day we boarded a small bus to explore the mountain and search for herbs. As we drove higher and higher, we passed through several bio-spheres. There has been much deforestation at the lower elevations on the North Korean side of the mountain, but on the Chinese side the forest is ancient and remains almost unaltered. The pristine forests are mainly pine at the lower elevations, but as you ascend the mountain, mountain birch trees predominate. The area is also well known as a natural habitat for deer, tigers, leopards, wolves, bears, and wild boars. I felt that I was in one of the wildest places I'd ever been.

As we rose higher and higher on the mountain, we were driving on dirt roads that sometimes became quite rough. Suddenly, we would come upon a place where the road had totally caved in and a huge puddle was blocking the way. We stopped at several Ginseng and Reishi farms to take photos and shoot video, but Ron was searching for something very special.

Every so often, we would see little old men come out of the woods and stand next to the road while holding out something in their hands. Ron explained that these men roam the forests looking for wild herbs, like Ginseng roots, and then wrap them in wet moss to keep the roots fresh. Every time that Ron saw one of these men standing by the roadside he'd tell the bus driver to stop. We'd all pile out of the bus and I would video Ron bargaining with the sellers. By the time the afternoon was over, Ron had acquired an excellent collection of very old wild Ginseng roots that he would take back to Los Angeles to make one of his rare connoisseur grade Ginseng tinctures.

At one point, we stopped where Schizandra grew wild. Ron fashioned a crown of wild Schizandra and placed it on his wife Yanlin's head to wear. She reminded me of Magu, so I took photos of her looking like a Nature Goddess. We all ate wild Schizandra, the herb that Ron's Daoist teacher, Master Park, considered the ultimate herb in all the world. I savored this special moment, high on sacred Changbai Mountain.

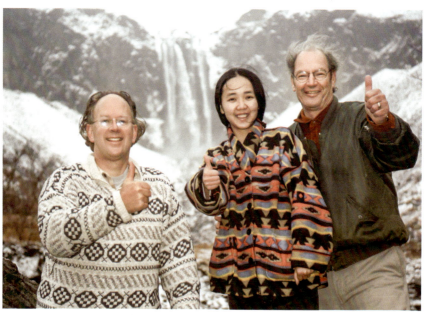

Ganga, Yanlin, and Ron at the Changbai Mountain waterfall

When we stopped at the Changbai waterfall, the air was filled with negative ions and I felt that I was breathing in the purest Chi (prana) that I'd ever experienced in my entire life. Above us was the towering 223-foot-tall waterfall, that flowed from Heaven Lake, and below us were hot springs where Chinese women would hard boil eggs for you. We could have stayed there forever, but we were on a mission.

We were looking for the best Reishi ever grown on Changbai Mountain. Someone had told Ron about this farm, but the bus driver couldn't find it. It was getting later and later in the afternoon, and if we didn't find it fast we'd be late getting down the mountain and would miss our flight back to Beijing. Ron finally said that we only had a half hour window, and if we didn't find the Reishi farm by then we'd have to give up the search. No one wanted to do that. We'd come so far, and to give up now would be a big disappointment.

There was a tremendous sense of urgency, and I began praying that we would find the Reishi farm and not return empty-handed. Suddenly, the bus driver announced that he had found it and pulled over in front of the farm. Ron and Yanlin jumped out of the bus and began running toward the Reishi tents. I quickly grabbed my camera gear and raced after them. As I was rushing to catch up with them, I heard Yanlin scream, "Oh my God, it's the best Reishi I've ever seen." I entered a long tent full of Reishi and saw Ron walking amidst hundreds of gorgeous reddish brown Reishi Mushrooms. There were many tents and each was filled with many hundreds of Reishi Mushrooms, growing on logs partly buried in the earth. I knew that we were pressed for time, but I rushed around from tent to tent taking photos of Ron inspecting the beautiful Reishi, known throughout the history of China as the King of Herbs.

We were introduced to Mrs. Mao, the scientist who ran the farm, and I videoed the conversation between her and Ron while Yanlin translated. She explained that they were cultivating Duanwood Reishi by inoculating logs of very aggressive wood with Reishi spores and that the resulting mushrooms were extremely potent. Much scientific research has been done on Reishi and the Japanese use Duanwood Reishi in cancer treatments because when used in conjunction with chemotherapy the patients have less negative side-effects from the chemotherapy.

Ron agreed to purchase the entire crop and the next year's crop as well. He had found what he was looking for—the best Reishi in the world. Mrs. Mao had the workmen gather some of the most exceptionally large mushrooms for us to take with us. I photographed Yanlin with the largest reishi they found. What a sight that was! We boarded the bus and began the long journey back to Beijing and finally Los Angeles. As I flew back to America, I felt that I had just been to the most amazing place I'd ever visited. When we got back home to the herbarium in Los Angeles, I told Ron, "Now I get it. Dragon Herbs is the storefront of Changbai Mountain." Ron gave me a knowing look, smiled and said, "I like that."

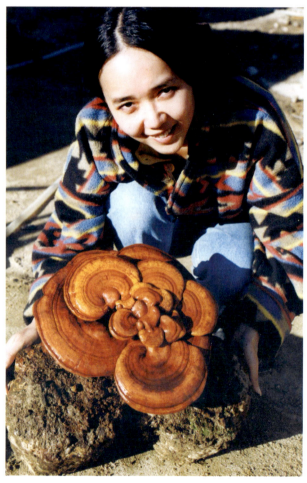

Yanlin Teeguarden with a beautiful Duanwood Reishi from Changbai Mountain

15. ENCOUNTERS WITH NOTABLE PEOPLE

I have friends who really dislike Los Angeles. They say things like, "If I ever have to go to Los Angeles, I stay one night and leave as fast as I can the next day." My experience of Los Angeles is very different. I've lived there three different times in my life, and each of those times were some of the absolute best periods of my life. Los Angeles is a powerful vortex of creative energy populated by artists of every kind as well as many very spiritually conscious people. I've made wonderful friends in Los Angeles and have encountered many very interesting people.

As my apprenticeship with Master Daoist Herbalist Ron Teeguarden continued, I noticed a blossoming of my heart, resulting in increased compassion that brought me into contact with people who I could help. I had always felt empathy for those who were suffering, but the compassion that I felt began to increase exponentially and it led me to rather miraculously encounter people who I could be of service to. A previous spiritual teacher took me aside one day and said, "You have a special ability to meet famous people. You should use it for the Dharma."

Two such people were Alanis Morissette and Joni Mitchell. I had read interviews with both Alanis and Joni in which they spoke frankly about extreme challenges they were facing. In Alanis' case, she mentioned how after she achieved the success she had always dreamed of, following the astronomical success of her album *Jagged Little Pill,* she still wasn't happy. The bleak reality that commercial success beyond her wildest dreams still didn't make her happy plunged her into a deep depression, and she even considered suicide. *Jagged Little Pill* had become one of the best-selling albums of all time, selling over 33 million units worldwide. Alanis had been striving for success ever since childhood, but now she found that fame and fortune didn't provide the happiness she had dreamed of.

As I read her honest and heartfelt confession of deep depression, I felt a wave of sympathy arise in my heart, and I wanted to do whatever I could to relieve her suffering. I had already experienced the personal effects of Shen tonics. These herbs, such as Wild Asparagus Root, Albizzia Flower, Spirit Poria, Wild Reishi, and Tibetan Rhodiola, stabilize and elevate the emotions. I had seen these Shen tonics do wonders with other people, and I felt that Alanis could benefit especially from a tonic formula known as Supreme Shen Drops.

I knew that Alanis lived in Santa Monica, only a few miles away from Ron's herbarium, so I decided to put a copy of Ron's book *The Ancient Wisdom of Chinese Tonic Herbs* in the trunk of my car in case I ever crossed paths with her. The book sat in my car for several months, but I knew that one day I would eventually meet Alanis. That day came when I went to the Bodhi Tree bookstore with my friend Larry. We were browsing for books when Larry came over to me and said, "Do you know who is over there?" I looked across the room, and to my surprise there was Alanis. My first thought was that now I could give her Ron's book. Then I realized that Larry had driven us, but fortunately the Bodhi Tree carried Ron's book, so I bought a copy and gave it to Alanis. She accepted it graciously with a big smile.

Amazingly, I ran into Joni Mitchell within a week. Again I was with Larry, having lunch at the Daily Grill in Brentwood. Larry whispered, "Look who is behind you at the next table." I glanced over my shoulder, and there was Joni Mitchell. Again, Larry had driven us, so I didn't have my car with Ron's book in the trunk. But we were only a short distance from Ron's herbarium, so I called a coworker and asked her to bring over a copy of Ron's book. I introduced myself to Joni and gave her the book. A few weeks later, I was brewing teas at the herbarium when I heard the front doorbell ring and in walked Joni Mitchell. She had a consultation, began taking several tonic formulas, and experienced a profound improvement from a combination of Jing, Chi, and Shen tonics. So, within a week I ran into both Alanis and Joni, two artists that I respected highly and wanted to assist in whatever way I could.

Another day, I went for lunch at a Brazilian restaurant in Brentwood. To my amazement, the Gracie family was there, wearing Gracie Jujitsu t-shirts. The Gracie family are recognized around the world as a dominant force in Mixed Martial Arts. I introduced myself to the father of the Gracie clan, told them that I worked for a world famous herbalist, and invited them to all come over to Ron's herbarium. They gladly accepted, and when they met with Ron, he showed them several tonic formulas that many athletes use to strengthen bones and ligaments. In particular, Cordyceps is an excellent herb that many Olympians use to improve athletic performance. It's a drug-free way to improve the lungs, increase muscle power, and gain greater endurance. As Ron explained the many benefits of Chinese Tonic Herbs for athletes, I brewed delicious tonic elixirs for the whole Gracie crew, and then they left with bags of herbal formulas.

One of the most memorable and surprising encounters that I had took place one night when I attended a lecture in Santa Monica. I had seen a flyer advertising a talk by a Yaqui Indian shaman, known as Grandfather Cachora, who was also an herbalist. The event was held in a small house in Santa Monica that was devoted to natural health and healing.

Grandfather Cachora was a short man with a super-powerful presence. He was very charismatic and had a radiant glow about him. My only knowledge of Yaqui traditions had come from reading all the Carlos Castaneda books. During the question and answer period, someone asked about Grandfather Cachora's relationship with Castaneda. He replied that Castaneda had created a fictional character named Don Juan that he had based on information which he had acquired from three different Yaqui shamans. Cachora said that, of the three, Castaneda had spent more time with him than the other two and that only the first book, *The Teachings of Don Juan: A Yaqui Way of Knowledge,* published in 1968, contained authentic Yaqui teachings. He said that after the first book, Carlos began making stuff up. I am not confirming or denying this version of the story because I have no first-hand knowledge of these events. All that I know is what I heard from Cachora and those around him.

When the event was over, I went up and introduced myself. Grandfather Cachora would have been over 80 at the time, and yet his face was smooth and when I shook his hand it felt as soft as a baby. I asked Cachora if he would like to visit my herbal master's herbarium, and he said that even though it was late, he could come right then. I called Ron to inform him that I was a bringing a Yaqui shaman over to the house who just might be the real Don Juan. Although Ron had already gone to bed, he was happy to meet Grandfather Cachora. Cachora has extensive knowledge of herbs, so it was a meeting of like minds. Ron showed Cachora many rare and exotic herbs and gifted Cachora with Reishi Mushrooms as well as many other herbs to take with him back to Mexico.

Later, we contacted Grandfather Cachora in Mexico and invited him to return to give a two-day workshop at Ron's herbarium. September 23rd was a beautiful autumn night and the talk by Cachora was attended by about 75 people, including Rosanna Arquette and Joni Mitchell. It turned out that Joni had read every book by Castaneda several times.

Cachora spoke in Spanish while Concepcion Laura translated. "Hola! Aloha! I am the guardian of the Mother Earth, guardian

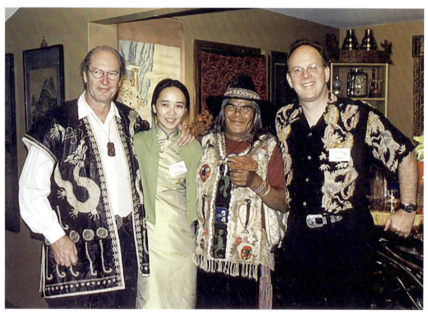

Ron, Yanlin, Grandfather Cachora, and Ganga

of the three kingdoms of the great medicine. I am a walker who goes amongst the unknown. My way is red—the red path—all the beings of Nature and the Heart of Humanity. I am an enemy of contamination, of smog—of any abuse to Mother Earth. My knowledge comes from the father and the mother. I know 4,000 medicinal plants, their purpose, what time to harvest them and during what moon, and what area to find them in."

The following day, Cachora offered a workshop in the back yard. He told us that his mother's ancestry was Mongolian and his father was Mayan. So Cachora himself was the product of East meeting West, and he carried two powerful bloodlines. Later, my wife Tara and I began going down to Mexico to visit Grandfather Cachora and take sweatlodges. My favorite memory is walking with Grandfather Cachora through his large garden while he lovingly watered every tree, plant, and flower. They were obviously his friends.

What I learned from these experiences is that we should treat every interaction with each person we meet in life as an opportunity to offer the best of who we are and what we have to offer. The Tibetan

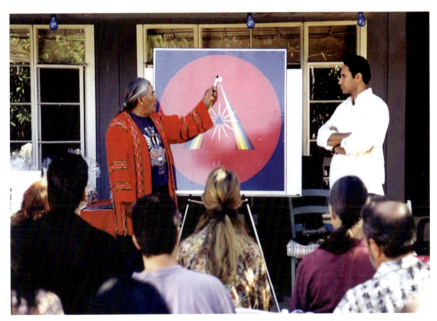

Grandfather Cachora teaching at Ron Teeguarden's home

Buddhists teach that we have all had so many lifetimes that every person on Earth has been our mother at some time. I actually don't know for sure if that is true, but I do know that every meeting is significant, and we can offer our best to everyone we meet.

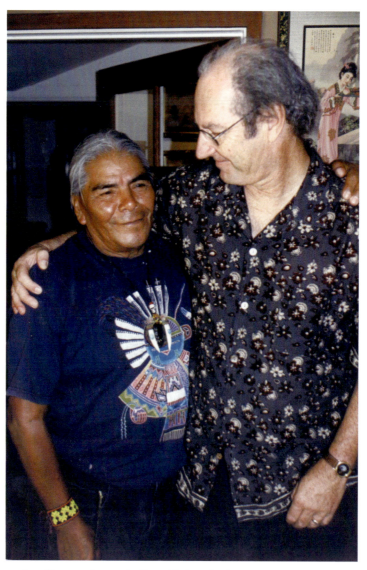

Ron Teeguarden with Grandfather Cachora in the herbarium

16. SEVEN YEARS IN INDIA

Just as the universe had led me to become the apprentice of Master Daoist Herbalist Ron Teeguarden, one day it led me in another direction.

One night, I gave a lecture in Los Angeles on "Herbs for Spiritual Development" and afterwards invited everyone who attended the talk to come over to Ron Teeguarden's herbarium, which was only about a mile away. As fate would have it, Tara, my current wife, was one of the people who attended the talk that night and then came over to the herbarium. Tara and I eventually moved to Del Mar and became the personal attendants of a Tibetan Buddhist teacher named Dzogchen Khenpo Choga Rinpoche. We served as his personal attendants for nearly three years, organized his Dharma teaching events, and helped him start his organization in America. Khenpo Choga was a rare lama who had been trained in Tibet, not in exile as had many of the Tibetan teachers currently teaching in the West. He was one of the greatest living Tibetan scholars and a highly accomplished yogi, who had completed a seven year cave retreat in the mountains of Tibet. Tara and I devoted ourselves to serving him and spent literally every dollar we had on helping start his spiritual organization.

Then, life again led us in a new direction. We met a beautiful Chinese woman teacher named Yuan Miao, who carried a Tibetan Dakini lineage. Within a day of meeting her, she invited us to move in to her foundation's house. For the next three years, we served her in the same way that we had Khenpo Choga, by organizing teaching tours for her and assisting in the establishment of her spiritual non-profit organization, the New Century Foundation. We would have stayed with Yuan Miao for the rest of our lives, being very content to help her with her mission, but one day she pushed us out of the nest, telling us that we had guru karma of our own and a mission to fulfill in the world.

In 2006 we decided to move to India and lived there for the next seven years. At that point, we had already been on the spiritual path for over thirty years and had been teaching meditation for over twenty years, but we felt that we had been swimming in the shallow end of the pool. We were guided to dive deep into the ancient spiritual traditions of India, specifically the Siddha tradition. The word "siddha" is a Sanskrit word that means a "perfected one" or "one who has attained the perfection of consciousness."

After about two and a half years of living in India, something rather dramatic happened. It was like a doorway opened and divine grace rained down upon us. We began to have the kind of inner experiences that we had read about in books like *Autobiography of a Yogi* by Paramahansa Yogananda, *The Play of Consciousness* by Swami Muktananda, and *Living with the Himalayan Masters* by Swami Rama. In addition to these inner experiences of consciousness, we also began having amazing experiences in the outer sphere of life when we would encounter, with no effort on our part, beautiful masters who bestowed great blessings upon us.

As the years in India passed, we met many amazing living masters and studied the lives of many more historical ones. We learned that many of these masters had attained tremendous longevity, along with what many would consider "supernatural abilities." However, these powers were not at all "supernatural," because they were actually the natural abilities of humans who were using the full potential of consciousness.

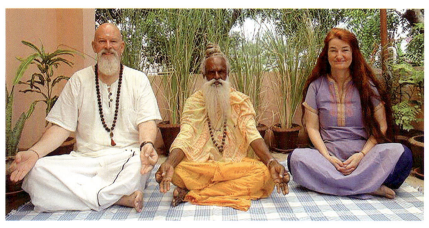

Ganga, Thirumoola Siddha Swami, and Tara

As we researched the lives of these great Siddha saints, we came to the conclusion that these Siddhas were Universal, not restricted to any religious, cultural, or geographic boundaries. In India they were called Siddhas. In Tibet, they were often called Mahasiddhas, or Great Siddhas, and in China they were known as the Daoist Immortals. As we studied each of these groups, we saw that all three had several things in common. They were experts in herbs and knew how to use herbs to cure any human ailment. They also were experts in alchemy, and finally all three groups knew how to attain tremendous longevity.

After four years of living continuously in India, without ever returning to America, we decided that it was time to begin sharing what we had experienced and learned in India. We felt that while we lived in India for all those years, we were like sponges soaking up the wisdom of India, and now the time had come to wring out the sponge and share what we had learned. We returned to America in 2010, with ninety dollars to our name and no car. Our dream was to travel for three months around America and give around fifty free seminars on the "Secrets of the Siddhas." The events were so popular that we ended up traveling for ten months and gave over one hundred and fifty free events to over three thousand people. We felt passionately that it was vital for the survival of humanity that people around the world understand about the lives of the great Siddha Saints. The world today is faced with many very serious problems: climate change, shortages of food, lack of clean water, war, and terrorism. In order to solve these problems, humanity must rise to a higher level of consciousness. The experts on raising consciousness are the Siddha Saints because they succeeded in accomplishing it themselves. They are humanity's greatest resource. Tara and I decided to devote the rest of our lives to educating the world about the Siddha Saints in order to contribute however we could to raising the consciousness of humanity.

17. MASTERS OF LONGEVITY

Many of the great Siddhas (perfected beings) of India, Tibet, and China lived extremely long lives. During the seven years that we lived in India, we learned of many great Siddhas and Mahasiddhas (Great Siddhas) who achieved tremendous longevity. One such enlightened master was Tapaswiji Maharaj. His life story is one of the most amazing in the long history of India. It is worth repeating here because it sheds light on the use of herbs to extend life.

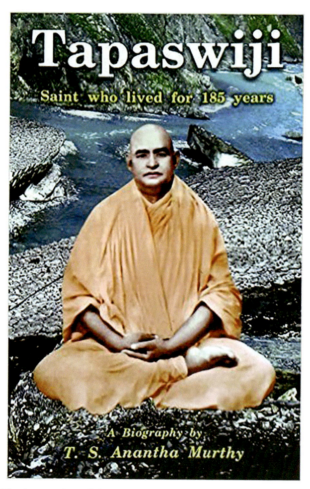

The biography of Tapaswiji—the Saint who lived 185 years by T.S. Anantha Murty

Tapaswiji was a king, a Maharaja, who had a palace in Maharashtra, in northwestern India. When he was fifty years old, his kingdom was under attack, so he had to go fight a war to defend his kingdom. When he returned to his palace, his wife, son, and brother were all dead. This plunged him into deep despair. Tapaswiji decided to ride his horse to Delhi to meet with the sultan who ruled that part of India. He wanted to ask the sultan to protect his kingdom, but the sultan offered him very unexpected advice. The sultan told Tapaswiji that it was more important to be concerned with knowing God than it was to be concerned with worldly affairs. When Tapaswiji left Delhi to return home, he was in a state of confusion.

Instead of returning to his palace, Tapaswiji headed to Haridwar—the Gateway to the Himalayas. There he found a God-realized guru and became his disciple. After twelve years, he had achieved the goal of yoga, union with God. Now that he had attained the goal of yoga, his guru told him to go deep into the Himalayas and to practice tapas (austerities). He did that for the next forty years, which is why he is known as Tapaswiji. He could meditate so well that he would find a suitable cave, sit down, go into samadhi (a superconscious state beyond thought), and two or three years would pass. Eventually, after forty years of doing tapas high in the Himalayas, Tapaswiji was a very aged 102-year-old man. He had lost his hair and his teeth, was very wrinkled, and had lost his flexibility from sitting in meditation for long stretches of time in cold caves. He decide that it was time, as they say in India, to "drop the body," but he had one last desire. He wanted to see the ocean before he died. People had always told him how beautiful the ocean is, how the blue stretches on forever, and how you can't see its limits. So, he decided to walk over a thousand miles, all the way from the Himalayas to Burma, to see the ocean.

On his way to Burma, Tapaswiji passed through Assam. There was a temple on a hill, and when he reached the temple, the priest asked him where he was going. Tapaswiji told the priest that he was going to Burma to see the ocean, and then he was going to drop the body. The priest told him that it sounded like a good idea, but he had another suggestion. He said that he had an herbal formula called Kaya Kalpa that traditionally was used to extend the lives of great saints, so that they could continue to be of service to humanity. The priest recognized that Tapaswiji was a great saint and offered the herbal formula to him. The only requirement was that he had to stay in a totally dark room for three months and all he could eat was the Kaya Kalpa herbal paste and drink fresh cow's milk. This was no problem for Tapaswiji. After all, he could sit in samadhi for the entire three months, so he agreed. At the conclusion of the three months, when he left the dark room, Tapaswiji had been rejuvenated back to how he had been when he was fifty years old. He had grown a new head of black hair, a new set of teeth, had lost his wrinkles, and had regained his vitality. This happened when Tapaswiji was 102 years old, and he went on to take the Kaya Kalpa two more times and lived to be 185 years old.

It is important to realize that this story is not a myth. Tapaswiji was a historical figure whose dates of birth and death are well documented. There was even an article in Life Magazine about Tapaswiji's long life and how he gave the Kaya Kalpa to two other famous individuals in India. Tapaswiji Maharaj died in 1955 at the age of 185.

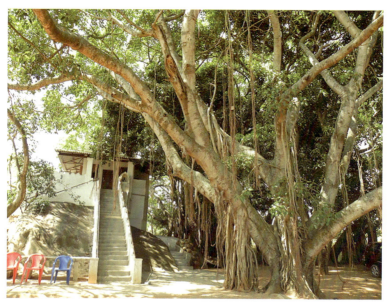

Tapaswiji's Ashram outside of Bangalore,
where he took the Kaya Kalpa the last two times

When Tara and I were living in India, we met and became friends with a man who was Tapaswiji's sanyasi disciple and who administered the Kaya Kalpa to Tapaswiji the last two times that he took it. One day this disciple of Tapaswiji asked us to help him bury three canisters of the Kaya Kalpa formula that needed to remain in the ground for forty-one days. It was a great honor to assist him in this important activity.

There are many such stories of great masters in India, Tibet, and China who, through the use of herbs, meditation, and spiritual practices, attained tremendous longevity. These great souls are living proof that we all can enjoy long lifespans of health, happiness, and spiritual fulfillment.

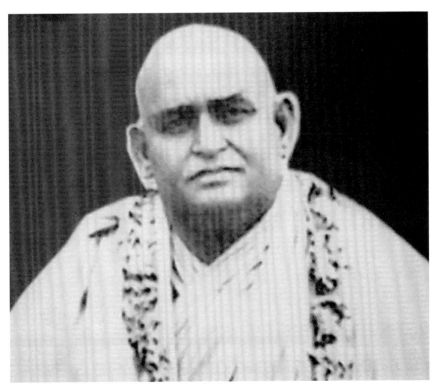

Tapaswiji Maharaj

18. RETURNING TO CHINA WITH RON AND YANLIN

It had been several years since I had seen my Daoist Herbal Master, Ron Teeguarden. During the years that I had been his apprentice and lived with his family, he had influenced my life profoundly. I missed him like a long-lost brother. When Tara and I returned to Los Angeles from India, Ron invited us over to his house for tea one day. We sat in his office beneath huge Tibetan thankas and he told us about his recent trip to Bhutan. It was an amazing story. As I listened to him, I remembered how wonderful it had been traveling with him to Changbai Mountain. When Ron finished telling us about his experiences in Bhutan, I said, "Ron, if you ever need one of your expeditions documented with video and photographs, we'd love to do it." I was shocked when he replied, "Would you really do that for me?" I thought, "Of course we would, in a heartbeat." Ron said that he was planning a trip to the original Shaolin temple in China for the coming year and that he'd love to have us document it. Wow, my inner being was jumping for joy. There was nothing I'd rather do than accompany Ron to China again.

After completing a teaching tour of America, Tara and I returned to India. Our life at that time was split between living in South India for six months of the year and then, when our visa was about to expire, we'd return to America to teach across the country. This time, however, we decided to not just teach across America but to teach all the way around the world. We left India and taught in Malaysia for a month. I emailed Ron from Kuala Lumpur and told him that we were on our way to Hong Kong to teach and that we could meet him in Beijing on August 1st. He replied that it was perfect timing because he was arriving in Beijing also on August 1st, and he'd meet us there. Then, he wrote, "I hope you don't mind. A few other people want to come on the trip, Rev. Michael Beckwith of Agape International Spiritual Center in Los Angeles and Gabriel Cousens of the Tree of Life Healing Center in Arizona." We were overjoyed. We knew of both of these men's life work and held them in high regard. It would be a joy traveling as a group to the Shaolin Temple.

After teaching in Hong Kong, Tara and I flew to Beijing and rendezvoused with Ron and his party. Ron had planned that on the first day we'd visit two very important places in Beijing. The first was the White Cloud Temple, which is the oldest Daoist temple in Beijing.

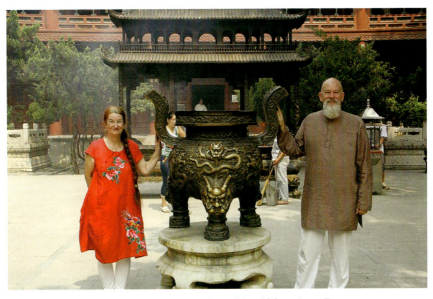

Tara and Ganga at the White Cloud Temple in Beijing

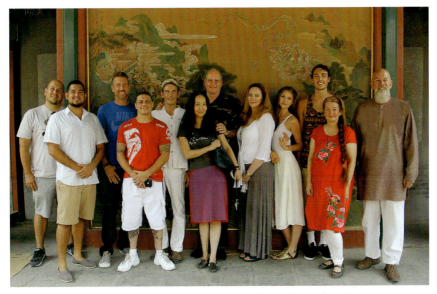

Ron, Yanlin, and friends at the White Cloud Temple in Beijing

The White Cloud Temple is said to have been built in AD 739 and was once the most influential Daoist temple in China. It was a very profound experience to walk where thousands of Daoists had walked in ancient times. At one point, I entered a temple where Ron was making incense offerings, and I couldn't help wonder if I had known him there in a past life. During our tour of the temple, Ron showed us a beautiful large mural that included Reishi Mushrooms.

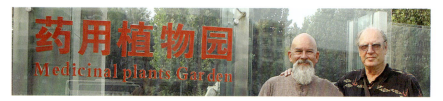

Ganga and Ron at the Beijing Medicinal Plant Garden

Our second stop in Beijing was the Institute of Medicinal Plant Development (IMPLAD). IMPLAD and Beijing Medicinal Plant Garden, affiliated with the Chinese Academy of Medical Sciences (CAMS), plays a leading role in research on Chinese medicinal herbs. The 667 staff, include 178 professors and associate professors.

Ron led us on a tour of the Medicinal Plant Garden, which is a huge botanical garden with just about every herb that grows in

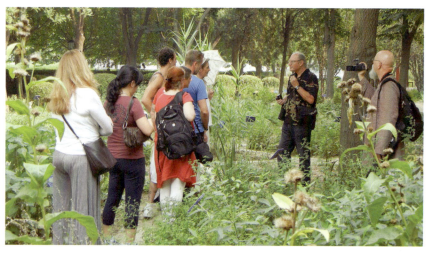

Ron explaining the properties of herbs in the Beijing Medicinal Plant Garden

China. I shot video of Ron speaking about many of the herbs. It was a wonderful experience to listen to a Master Daoist Herbalist explain the properties of many of the finest herbs in the world. Afterwards, we were treated to a lunch that consisted of entirely Tonic Herbs. I remarked that it was the best meal that I ever ate and that I wished that I could eat meals of only Tonic Herbs every day of my life.

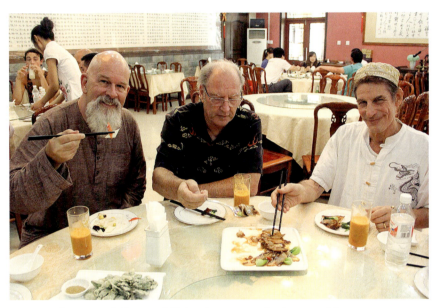

Ganga with Ron and Gabriel, enjoying the best meal I ever ate

I couldn't help but think that our health would be greatly improved if we could eat a diet that consisted of mostly or all Tonic Herbs. As we savored this delicious meal, Tara and I mentioned to Ron that we'd like to teach classes in Cooking With Tonic Herbs. After all, people in China have been cooking with the Tonic Herbs for thousands of years. They include the Tonic Herbs in their soups and stews because they understand that the Superior Herbs develop good health by increasing vitality, nurturing the Three Treasures, and producing a calm mind with a peaceful heart. Maybe we can learn a lot about how to eat in harmony with Natural Laws. We can all learn how to cook with Tonic Herbs and teach others how to do the same.

19. PILGRIMAGE TO THE SHAOLIN TEMPLE

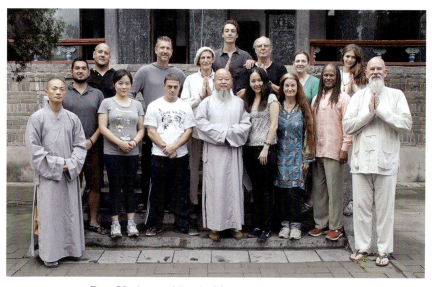

Ron, Yanlin, and Lucky Teeguarden with friends
who accompanied them on a pilgrimage to the Shaolin Temple

On our second day in Beijing, we were to all to meet in the morning at Ron and Yanlin's hotel and then fly from Beijing to Luoyang which is about sixty kilometers from the Shaolin Temple. When I woke up that morning, I could hardly believe that soon we'd be on our way to the famous Shaolin Temple that had played such an important role in my spiritual life. In our youth, both Tara and I had been dedicated watchers of the TV show "Kung Fu," starring David Carradine. Those readers who had the same experience know exactly what I mean. Those who never watched "Kung Fu" will have to imagine what an impact it had on young Americans who knew nothing of Eastern culture. I remember being completely absorbed in every episode of the show, which was based on the life of a monk from the Shaolin Temple. Having grown up on a media diet of the Mickey Mouse Club and Howdy Doody, "Kung Fu" was our first introduction to the Wisdom of the East.

As we rode on the bus from Luoyang to the Shaolin Temple,

memories of "Kung Fu" flashed through my mind. "Kung Fu" followed the adventures of Kwai Chang Caine, a Shaolin monk traveling through the American Old West, armed only with his spiritual training from the Shaolin Temple. Caine was a man of few words, but when he spoke, his dialogue was often based on aphorisms from the Dao De Ching, a book of ancient Daoist philosophy attributed to the sage Lao Tzu.

The TV show "Kung Fu" played a very important role in both Tara's and my spiritual path. It planted seeds in our consciousness that led

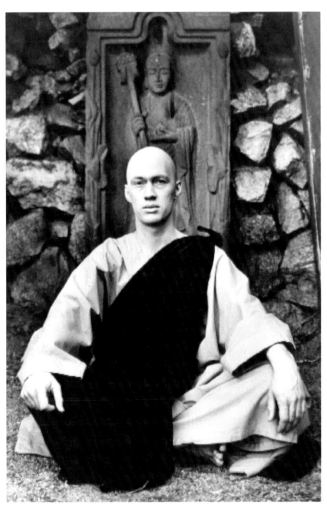

David Carradine as Kwai Chang Caine in the television show "Kung Fu"

us to where we are today. I often wonder if I would be the person that I am today if I hadn't watched "Kung Fu" in my youth. My intuition tells me that "Kung Fu" rekindled past life memories that Tara and I had as Daoist and Buddhist monks. Soon, we began reading books on Zen and Daoism by D.T. Suzuki, Alan Watts, and of course, Lao Tzu. As the decades passed, we continued on the spiritual path and explored many other wisdom traditions: Hinduism, Sufism, Native American, and Mystic Christianity. For the last seven years, we'd been living in India, deeply submerged in the complexity of Indian spirituality. So, in a sense, this trip to the Shaolin Temple with Ron, his wife Yanlin, Rev. Michael Beckwith, Gabriel Cousens, and a few other friends, represented a return to our roots. As we drew closer to the Shaolin Temple, the words kept going through my mind, "At this point in my life, Zen is the shoe that fits."

The Shaolin Temple is of great historic importance in the spiritual history of Asia. It is from the Shaolin Temple that not one but two great wisdom traditions flowed forth to benefit humanity. It is where the Indian Buddhist monk Bodhidharma meditated in a cave for nine years. Bodhidharma is credited as the founder of Zen and the creator of Kung Fu. The original name of Zen when it began in China was Chan, which was the Chinese way of pronouncing the Indian word "dhyana," which means "meditation." Chan eventually spread throughout China, Korea, and Japan. When it reached Japan, the Japanese pronounced Chan as Zen, and today much of the world knows it as Zen. Originally, Old Zen was devoid of ritual and dogma, but today it has become a religion and, like most religions, has accumulated rituals and dogma. But original Zen was simple. It was based on sitting, meditating, and becoming aware of your true nature. It is the direct experience of the true nature of mind, your Buddha Nature. Zen is called a sudden path to enlightenment, and the Shaolin Temple is where it all began with the monk Bodhidharma, known in China as Da Mo.

According to legend, Bodhidharma was an Indian prince who was the favorite son of the king. Bodhidharma had two jealous brothers who tried to kill him, but he had good karma and avoided their assassination attempts. Instead of entering into politics,

Bodhidharma became a Buddhist monk and a disciple of a wise Buddhist master, Prajñātāra. Bodhidharma studied under his master for many years. One day he asked Prajñātāra, "Master, when you pass away, where should I go? What should I do?" Prajñātāra replied to his devoted student that he should go to Zhen Dan, which was the name for China at that time. After Prajñātāra passed away, Bodhidharma left for China. It is said that Bodhidharma passed over many mountains and bodies of water on his way to China. Modern scholars date his arrival in China as the early fifth century.

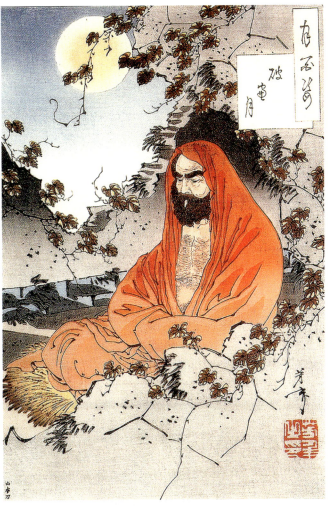

Bodhidharma (Da Mo), who meditated for nine years in a cave above the Shaolin Temple and who is credited with founding both Chan (Zen) and Kung Fu.

Eventually, Bodhidharma settled near the Shaolin Temple. After he had meditated for nine years in a cave on top of a mountain near the Shaolin Temple, the monks built him a room and invited him to come live in the monastery at the foot of the mountain. When he arrived, Bodhidharma noticed that the monks at the Shaolin Temple were in poor physical condition. The monks spent most of their time meditating and studying with little exercise. To remedy this, Bodhidharma instituted a system of physical conditioning that is now known throughout the world as Kung Fu.

We were provided with a monk named Li Bo who was our guide throughout our stay at the Shaolin Temple. As we entered the temple grounds, I was awestruck by the realization that I was walking where Bodhidharma and countless monks over many centuries had walked. We were not going to the Shaolin Temple as mere tourists. Ron had been invited by the abbot of the Shaolin Temple to discuss producing products based on ancient Shaolin Temple herbal formulas. Because we were guests of the abbot, we were allowed to enter areas of the temple that the public usually is not admitted to.

The Shaolin Temple's inside area is 160×360 meters, or 57,600 square meters. It has seven main halls on the central axis and seven other halls around, with several yards around the halls. The Shaolin Temple is full of outstanding examples of traditional Chinese architecture. If you are interested in Chinese traditional culture, it is a feast for the eyes. The amazing halls, temples, statues, and courtyards were beautiful to see, but for me there was another treasure to experience. I was acutely aware of the energetics of the place and how these buildings had housed hundreds of thousands of monks whose lives were dedicated to spiritual practice. As I walked through the many inspiring sights, I opened my heart to receive the blessings of these illumined practitioners of Zen and Kung Fu.

Some of the notable temple structures include:
  The Forest of Steles
  Ciyun Hall, including 124 stone tablets of various dynasties
  Heavenly Kings (Devaraja) Palace Hall
  Bell Tower (built in 1345; reconstructed in 1994)
  Drum Tower (built in 1300; reconstructed in 1996)

Kimnara Palace Hall
Six Patriarchs Hall
Mahavira Palace Hall (built around 1169; reconstructed in 1985)
Dhyana (Meditation) Halls
Dharma (Sermon) Hall
Standing in Snow Pavilion
Manjusri Palace Hall
Samantabhadra Palace Hall
White Robe (Avalokitesvara) Palace Hall (built in Qing dynasty)
Ksitigarbha Palace Hall (built in early Qing dynasty)
1000 Buddha Palace Hall (built in 1588; repaired in 1639,1776)
Bodhidharma Pavilion (built first in the Song dynasty)

As you enter the temple grounds, you walk along a pathway that is lined with inscriptions on stone steles that were made during several different dynasties. Ron pointed out to us very old trees that had many holes in the trunks. He explained that over centuries Shaolin monks had thrust their fingers into the trunk to develop their ability to project Chi power. As I put my fingers into the holes, I thought of all the monks before me who had done the same, and I wondered if perhaps I had been one of them in a past life.

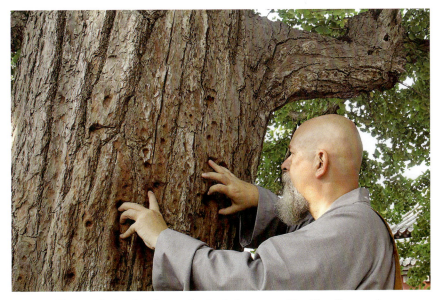

Ganga placing his fingers in the holes created by Shaolin monks

One afternoon, Ron showed Tara and me the Forest of Pagodas Yard, which was built before 791. It has 240 tomb pagodas of various sizes from the Tang, Song, Jin, Yuan, Ming, and Qing dynasties (618–1911). This is a graveyard for many of the most illustrious Buddhist Masters associated with the Shaolin Temple throughout the ages. The Masters are entombed in pagodas that average about 50 feet high. The form of each pagoda reflects the Master's status and attainment. The Shaolin Temple Pagoda Forest complex is the largest in all of China. As Ron pointed out especially unique pagodas, it was

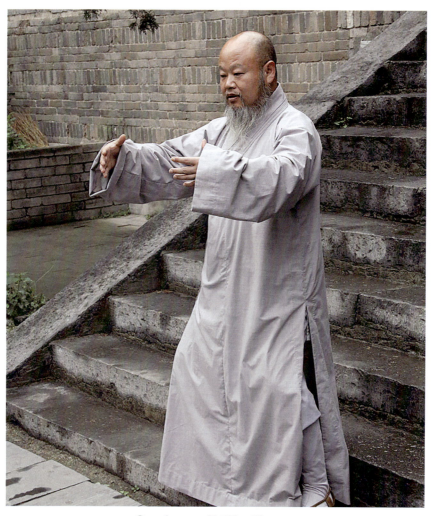

Grandmaster Shi Yan Zhuang,
head of all martial arts training at the Shaolin Temple

humbling to think that we were walking among the remains of many exemplary Buddhist practitioners and highly realized spiritual beings.

One of the highlights of our pilgrimage to the Shaolin Temple was that we were given personal Qigong instruction by Shifu Shi Yan Zhuang, the Master of all Martial Arts at the Shaolin Temple. He was an imposing figure who possessed a powerful presence. I felt incredibly honored to be able to have personal instruction from someone as advanced as Shifu Shi Yan Zhuang. It was truly a humbling experience. Obviously this was not something that happened for every tourist who visits the temple. We were being given special treatment because Ron had been invited by the abbot.

Our guide, Li Bo, gave us an impressive demonstration of Kung Fu. His strength, stamina, speed, and flexibility were truly astounding. Afterwards he gave us a class in the Eight Silken Brocades.

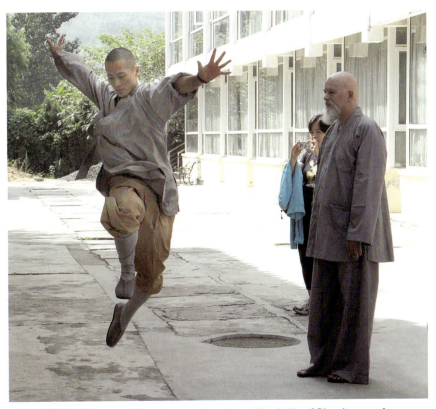

Li Bo demonstrating the amazing Kung Fu skills of Shaolin monks

Later, Li Bo showed us the stairs that go all the way to the Dharma Cave, where Bodhidharma sat in meditation for nine years. Because of their peak physical conditioning, the Shaolin monks can climb these stairs on all fours in the amazingly short time of 30 minutes. The cave is about 23 feet deep and 10 feet high, with many inscriptions carved in stone on both its sides. To visit this holy cave is to

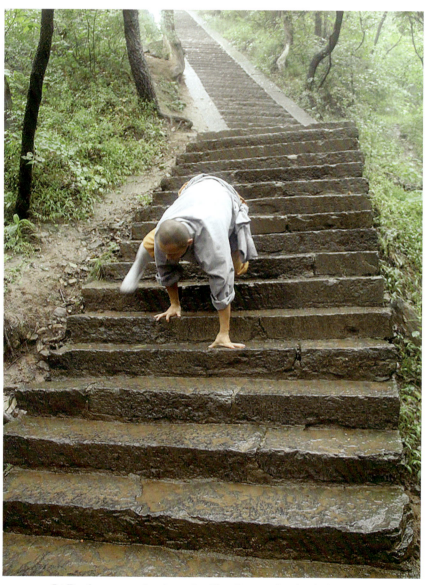

Li Bo demonstrating how the Shaolin monks climb the stairs

be where Zen Buddhism originated by virtue of Bodhidharma's perseverance in deep meditation. His shakti (energy) still permeates the stone walls of the cave.

The Shaolin Temple training combines Zen for cultivating the mind, Kung Fu for developing a strong and healthy body, and medical skills for health. On our final day at the Shaolin Temple, Ron invited us to accompany him to the Shaolin Pharmacy Bureau, where he was going to discuss developing herbal products based on ancient Shaolin formulas. As we entered the lobby, we saw an altar, and on that altar was a large Reishi Mushroom on one side and a large Chaga Mushroom on the other side. This was evidence of how highly revered Reishi and Chaga are at the Shaolin Temple.

One afternoon, while walking through the temple grounds, I noticed a tree with a beautifully curved trunk and felt an overwhelming urge to sit next to that old tree to meditate. As I sank deeper and deeper in meditation, images of Shaolin monks flashed within my mind. I thought of all the monks who had meditated here and felt profoundly blessed by all of them.

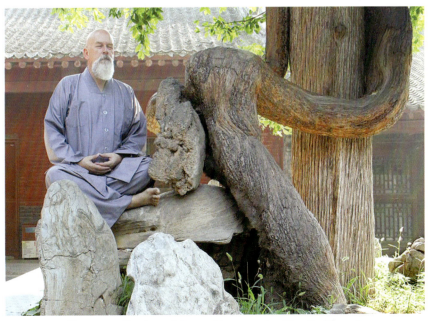

Ganga meditating with an old tree at the Shaolin Temple

On our final night, we were invited to attend a concert that we were told would include New Age music. To be honest, I didn't expect it to be more that a cheesy performance and really didn't want to go. I thought a better idea for our last night at the Shaolin Temple would be to stay in our hotel room and meditate. But the tickets were already purchased and, not wanting to appear rude, I went anyway. Boy, was I wrong. When we arrived at the concert, it was held in a giant outdoor amphitheater and the stage area was an entire mountainside. The sets, costumes, music, and lighting were all fantastic. When the concert ended, all of us in our party agreed that it was the most professional and spectacular production that we'd ever seen anywhere in the world. Many of us said that it would be worth the trip to China just to see it. So much for preconceptions.

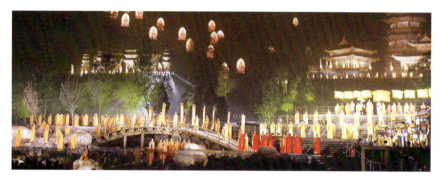

Theatrical presentation at the Shaolin Temple

The next morning we left the Shaolin Temple, filled with many beautiful memories and with a deep sense of gratitude that Ron and Yanlin had invited us on this pilgrimage to such a sacred spiritual realm. The trip to the Shaolin Temple had been a pivotal experience in our spiritual lives. We came home to Zen. Zen was indeed the shoe that fit.

20. THE SECRETS OF SPIRITUAL DEVELOPMENT

In China, throughout the ages, spiritual development was known as self-cultivation. Self-cultivation took many forms and had many aspects: diet, herbs, meditation, breathing techniques, and positive thinking and living habits. Modern people are always looking for a fast fix, but self-cultivation is not as simple as taking a few herbal capsules. To develop a truly healthy and fulfilled life requires taking a good hard look your lifestyle and making changes for the better.

During my time as Ron Teeguarden's apprentice, I witnessed many people who came through his herbarium and who experienced varying degrees of improvement. Some took the Tonic Herbs for a while, began to get benefits, and then stopped, slipping back to their previous state. Some took the Tonic Herbs, got benefits, but continued the bad habits that had caused their health problems in the first place. And then there were those who took the herbs regularly, received profound benefits, and made the conscious decision to alter their life-style to promote health and happiness.

One thing that I know for sure is that the Tonic Herbs work. About that I have no doubt. They have been time-tested for thousands of years with proven results and I have personally experienced those positive results myself. But if one is interested in attaining high states of consciousness, then they must be combined with sensible, beneficial, life-promoting habits. If someone persists in overworking, not getting enough sleep, eating an unhealthy diet, abusing drugs or alcohol, and allowing negative mental and emotional patterns to control their life, they will not be able to achieve lasting good health. Eventually they will develop health problems like exhaustion, hypertension, anxiety, and depression.

There is another way to live one's life. The ancient Daoist and Buddhist sages who were experts in Tonic Herbalism knew how to live according to Nature's Laws in order to experience great longevity and ultimately enlightenment. We can learn much from them.

Perhaps one of the most interesting of these Chinese herbalist sages was the legendary Li Qing Yun (1677-1933), who said that he was over 200 years old. His life story was reported in newspaper articles and historical records of his time. Li Qing Yun was a traditional Chinese doctor and herbal expert, but he was also a Qigong master who maintained a very healthy lifestyle. In May of 1933, Time magazine published an article entitled "Tortoise-Sparrow-Dog" about Li Qing Yun. This article explained his longevity secrets, which were to maintain a tranquil mind, sit like a turtle, walk like a sparrow, and sleep like a dog. For over two hundred years he spent his time collecting herbs in the mountains. This reminds me of Ron's teacher's teacher, Moo San Do Sha, who was also extremely old and spent his days walking on trails in the mountains of Korea, living entirely on Tonic Herbs.

Li Qing Yun stated that his good health and longevity were the result of three things: being a vegetarian, maintaining inner peace, and drinking Goji Berry tea. Most importantly, he was adamant that maintaining inner peace was essential for longevity. Li led a very regulated lifestyle. He abstained from hard liquor and cigarettes and ate at regular times. He was early to bed and early to rise. He would also sit in meditation for a few hours at a time. Li also conserved his energy by speaking little, and only when necessary.

Li's entire life was spent studying Chinese herbs. During his long life he traveled throughout China, collecting herbs and looking for the secrets of longevity. Li Qing Yun's extraordinary life span of over 200 years is evidence that he succeeded in this pursuit. His age may or may not be accurate, but certainly he lived an extremely long life, and we can learn much from how he lived his life. Few of us dream of living as long as Li Qing Yun, but we all would like to enjoy long, healthy, and fulfilled lives. By putting into practice some of the principles that Li Qing Yun and other great illumined masters lived by, we, too, can achieve lives worth living.

The Tonic Herbs are Nature's greatest treasures. They are powerful tools that can enable us to develop and maintain a state of Radiant Health.

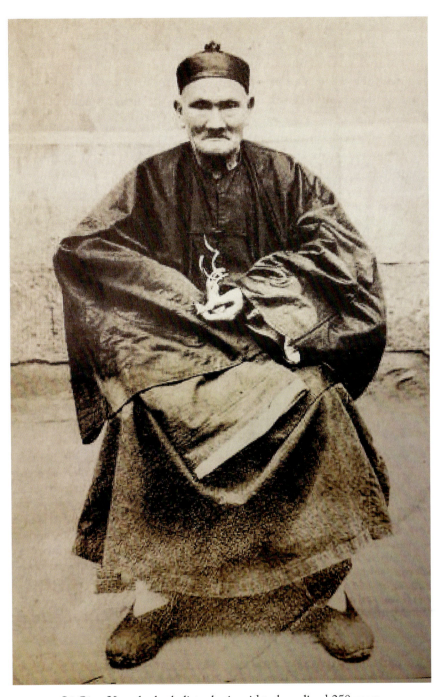

Li Qing Yun, the herbalist who is said to have lived 250 years.
The exact span of his life is not what is important.
What is important is what he taught about how to live a long and fulfilling life.

If we utilize these tools, combined with sensible habits such as a healthy diet, adequate rest and relaxation, meditation, eliminating bad habits that undermine our peace of mind and disrupt our physical health, we can achieve an uncommonly fine life. This is our birthright, but we must make wise choices in order to achieve it.

The Daoist and Buddhist sages were experts in health and longevity. Their lives were dedicated to self-cultivation and the attainment of enlightenment. We owe them all, both past and present, a debt of gratitude for they accumulated the knowledge that can enable us to live long lives and ultimately attain enlightenment. I sincerely wish that all of you reading this book take full advantage of these greatest treasures of Nature and achieve the pinnacle of human life. May all beings swiftly attain health, happiness, and full enlightenment.

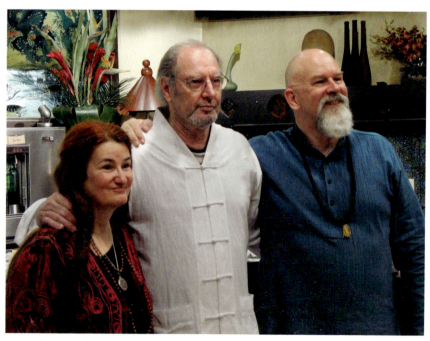

Ganga and Tara with Master Daoist Tonic Herbalist Ron Teeguarden

21. HOW TO TAKE TONIC HERBS

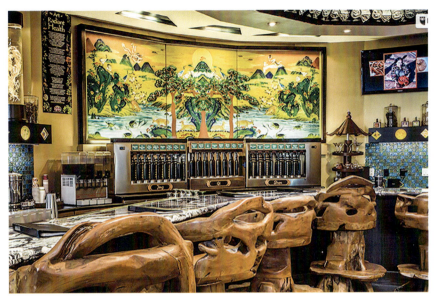

Dragon Herbs Herbal Emporium on Robertson Blvd in Beverly Hills

One of the first things that Ron told me when I became his apprentice was that "Compliance is the first rule of Tonic Herbalism." To put it simply, if you want to get the benefit from these wonderful herbs, you must take them. My personal experience has been that taking them regularly is very important. There is a rule in Tonic Herbalism that says that one should take them for three months in order to see improvement; however, I've seen hundreds of people notice benefits in a matter of weeks. Everyone is unique and responds differently.

There's a variety of ways that you can take the Tonic Herbs. There are capsules of spray dried powders, liquid tinctures, custom teas, and raw herbs. I personally use all four.

In the morning, afternoon, and evening, I have a cup of Spring Dragon Longevity Tea, which I believe is the most healthy tea in the world. I add to my cup of tea an eye dropper full of four tinctures: Goji and Schizandra Drops, 8 Immortals, Supreme Shen

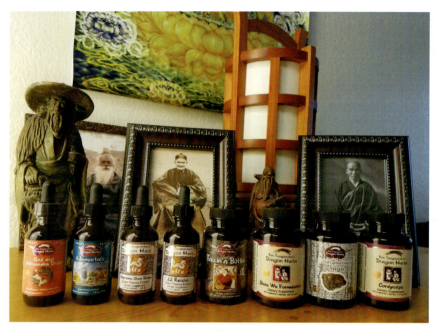

Ganga's Daily Herbal Program

Drops, and 22 Reishis. I also take two capsules of spray dried powders: Shou Wu Formulation, Tao in a Bottle, Chaga, and Cordyceps.

The products that I consider essential are Goji and Schizandra, 8 Immortals, Supreme Shen Drops, and Shou Wu Formulation. I take these every day of my life. I take the Chaga and Cordyceps just to give myself an extra boost of those supertonic herbs even though they are contained in some of the other tinctures.

For breakfast, my wife and I make a smoothie with Tonic Alchemy that contains 91 amazing ingredients. And, during the day, if I feel the need for a snack, I have some Heaven Mountain Goji Berries or Hermit's Mix. That's just my personal herbal routine that over time I've discovered works for me.

Another great way to take the Tonic Herbs is by using a Desktop Botanical Garden. These Glass Tea Elixir Makers are a great way to brew your own tonic herbal concoction, either on your desk at work or at home. They are made from non-reactive and non-porous glass that is perfect for extracting botanicals. There is no better way to get started as a budding herbalist than to start brewing your own elixirs yourself.

I'll share with you a practice that I have found very beneficial. This is just something that I do and is not required. It's totally optional, but I find that it enhances my consumption of Tonic Herbs. I view the Tonic Herbs as Nature's greatest gift to humanity. It is truly a miracle that Nature has produced such an abundance of plants that have so many beneficial effects on our health and well-being. I feel that it is entirely appropriate to express gratitude to the plants that have given their lives so that my life will be improved. So, before drinking my tea, smoothie, or swallowing capsules, I visualize the plants that have provided these healing substances and I thank them. Gratitude is important, and all too often we forget to express gratitude for all that we have been provided. Obviously, this is optional and not required to gain benefit from the Tonic Herbs. However, it works for me so I feel to pass it on to you, dear reader.

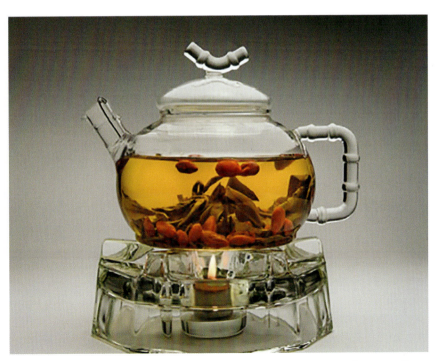

"The first rule of Tonic Herbalism is compliance."

22. MAKING IT EASIER FOR YOU TO START RECEIVING THE BENEFITS OF TONIC HERBS

Our intention in writing this book is to share the benefits of the Tonic Herbs with as many people as possible. We have experienced these profound benefits for many years and know first-hand how the Tonic Herbs can improve one's quality of life.

We have asked Ron Teeguarden to make it easier for you to begin receiving these benefits. Ron has graciously agreed to offer you a 10% discount on your first order from Dragon Herbs. Plus, you will also receive free shipping.

When you place your first order, just give them the code "gangatara" and they will give you the 10% discount. If you order online at the Dragon Herbs website (www.dragonherbs.com) just enter the "gangatara" code in the promotion code space.

When I started living with Ron's family and working as his apprentice, many of my friends asked how they could get started taking the Tonic Herbs. My advice is to have a free consultation from an herbalist trained by Ron Teeguarden. These free consultations are available by calling Dragon Herbs at (888) 558-6642. A senior herbalist will help you determine what kind of herbal program will best suit your needs. Herbal consultations from Dragon Herbs are always free.

Or, if you already know what herbs you are interested in, you can go to the Dragon Herbs website (www.dragonherbs.com) to review different products and then order either online or over the phone.

If you happen to live in the Los Angeles area, you can always stop in to one of the beautiful Dragon Herbs Emporiums and talk to a tonic herbalist in person.

We wish you health, happiness, longevity, and full enlightenment.

Ganga and Tara

22 TONIC HERBS BY TARA

Zhou Jing said:

"Jing, Qi, and Shen activate the human being.
If they are not depleted they will work intrinsically to produce
the substances needed to remain youthful. The ancients have stated:
'Heaven has three treasures: the sun, moon, and stars.
Mankind has three treasures: Jing, Qi, and Shen.'"

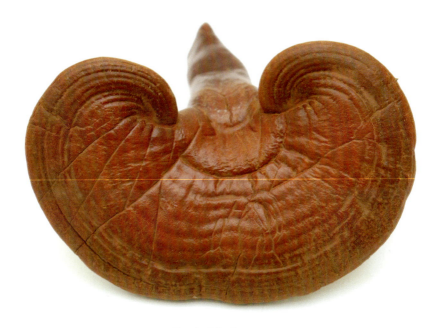

Reishi Mushroom

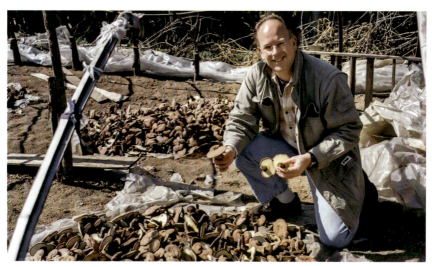

Ganga at a Duanwood Reishi farm on Changbai Mountain in China

1. REISHI

Ganoderma Lucidum, Ling Zhi

"Herb of Spiritual Potency"

Nourishes All Three Treasures: Jing, Chi, and Shen
Organ Meridians: Heart, Kidneys, Liver, Lungs
Spiritual Qualities: Opening of the Heart, Peacefulness, Mindfulness, Calmness, Willpower, Realization, Wisdom

Reishi Mushroom is the supreme Shen Tonic of all Chinese herbalism. Pronounced "Ling-Zhi" in China, this beautiful warm red mushroom has essentially been revered by the Chinese for thousands of years because of its incredible spiritual potency.

Paintings of the great Chinese Emperors often depicted them holding Reishi, as it was considered auspicious and all-powerful, even miraculous. Gods and Immortals were painted holding a staff like Lingzhi Mushroom. This sacred mushroom is often sculpted into pillars and painted in murals and other aspects of architecture. So highly was Reishi acclaimed that it became embedded in the culture through 5,000 years of civilization, leaving its imprint on medicine, religion, legend, literature, art, and architecture.

Sought after not only by the Emperors and the Royalty of China and Korea for longevity, but also by sages, Buddhist monks, and Daoists. Those true spiritual adepts sought Reishi not only for radiant health that would promise longevity, but as a means to hasten their spiritual enlightenment; and for a few, the possibility of Immortality.

Reishi's supreme power as an anti-stress herb was truly captured by the spiritual culture of Asia. Growing high in the mountains of Asia where spiritual adepts, hermits, monks, and Daoists naturally gravitated to do their spiritual cultivation, these Reishi Mushrooms offered support for practice. Monks and other adepts using these potent mushrooms found it easier calming the mind, releasing tension, building up their ability to focus, strengthening the nerves, sharpening their concentration, improving memory, and developing stronger willpower, all allowing for the cultivation of wisdom. Over time, Reishi became known as the "Mushroom of Spiritual Potency" by spiritual aspirants dependent on enduring long periods of focused physical, mental, and spiritual practices leading to flowering of spirit, wisdom, and enlightenment.

With such extensive impact on a civilization's health, culture, and spirituality, it's no wonder that Reishi became known as the "King of Herbs," the "Herb of Good Fortune," and the "Mushroom of Immortality."

What makes this herb so powerful and makes it a major longevity tonic? Reishi is among only a handful of herbs that are able to nourish all Three Treasures: Jing, Chi, and Shen. So in reality its potency is both in the physical and spiritual domain. It has a broad range of benefits that affect four major organs our life depends on: the Heart, Kidneys, Liver, Lungs.

Today Reishi's anti-stress support to the nervous system, mind, and memory improving ability, have all been supported by scientific research. This, along with its anti-inflammatory properties, immune modulating ability, it may prove to assist in a wide range of degenerative diseases of the elderly. Reishi is probably one of the most well-researched herbs in modern times, especially by the Japanese and Asian research community. In the future, it may become more prevalent in assisting those struggling with chemical dependencies and addictions.

Reishi is one of the most powerful natural adaptogens found on Earth. It is much more than an immune stimulant. It is an immune modulator that improves the immune system by regulating either deficient or excessive functions, meaning that it has double-direction activity, bringing those extremes into balance.

Let's look at some of its special abilities. Ganoderma Lucidum is more often known in the West by the Japanese name "Reishi." After much proven research, Reishi became used in Japan for healing certain cancers, as well as reducing side-effects from treatment by radiation and chemotherapy. Wild Ganoderma has been found to contain a substance called organic germanium, which the Japanese believe to have immune strengthening and anti-cancerous activity. Reishi also stimulates production of our bodies' own anti-cancer substance, which may prove it potentially to be one of the greatest cancer prevention substances. It has also been shown to protect one from radiation, especially if taken before irradiation.

Asians use this revered mushroom to improve the heart and cardiovascular system. In an age when cardiovascular conditions are so prevalent, angina, hardening of the arteries, and shortness of breath associated with cardiovascular disease can be prevented and treated with Reishi. General lowering of blood pressure is also achieved, balancing of cholesterol and thinning of the blood are all possible. Also, research in Japan and China has proven its ability to reverse leukopenia, the death of white blood cells.

Regarding lung conditions, Reishi is also useful in the curing and treatment of bronchitis; also potential treatment of allergies, hay fever, and bronchial asthma.

It also can be used to treat other allergic conditions and autoimmune disorders such as drug allergies, anaphylactic shock, and dermatitis. Especially effective in anti-allergic treatment of cell-mediated allergies, its anti-allergic activity has been identified as four triterpene ganodermic acids.

When considering liver stress and illnesses, Reishi is a highly effect treatment for hepatitis. It has been proven to have anti-hepatoxic activity, thereby promoting recovery of liver cells after surgery or physical injury.

Reishi's natural environment has been in Asian mountains: China, Korea, and Manchuria. In fact, though, they were also found thousands of years ago in the Americas by indigenous Native American tribes.

Shennong, the divine Farmer, stated there are at least six types of Reishis found, noted by their main color: Red, Purple, Black, White, Green, and Yellow. Each type affects a particular organ more than others. Purple Reishi has become extremely rare to find.

The two most prized forms are wild Red Reishi and Duanwood Reishi. The best Reishi is sought after in the mountainous regions of China and found growing wild on rotting trunks of indigenous hardwood trees. These days it is only the red and black Reishi that are commonly available. Ron says that the Duanwood Reishi is twice as potent as any other mushroom. It is grown on wood from the Duanwood tree, which enhances the medicinal properties of the mushroom.

Duanwood Reishi is now cultivated on Duanwood logs inoculated with their spores and planted in soil of pristine mountain areas or in the same environments, but contained in greenhouses. Ron Teeguarden rates these as excellent quality. They are grown without pesticides, as the mushrooms would die if pesticides were used on them, and thus they are thankfully protected by anti-pesticide laws.

Reishi Spores

Reishi Spores traditionally have been believed to produce an even more subtle and profoundly concentrated Shen Tonic than the fruiting caps alone.

Chinese and Japanese scientist have now proven that the spores have even more powerful immunological activity than the mushroom cap when technologically "cracked." Reishi Spores, the actual seed of the mushroom, have become known as the "Elixir of Life," a powerful Jing Tonic.

Reishi Spores must be processed in a special way to make their essence bioavailable to the human intestinal tract.

Reishi Mycelium

The mycelium of the Reishi Mushroom is the bulbous portion usually hidden from sight, but from which the sexual part, the fruiting reishi mushroom cap, grows. The mycelium is a powerful immune system stimulant.

It's important to remember that mycelium does not have the broad range of effect that the fruiting cap of the mushroom has, and should not be mistaken as a Shen tonic. You shouldn't buy mycelium thinking you are getting all the benefits you would expect from Reishi Mushroom. Important note: Reishi must be cooked to extract its essence; do not eat it raw.

Contraindications: None. Allergic reaction to Reishi is relatively nonexistent. Extremely high doses could cause sleepiness the first few times taken.

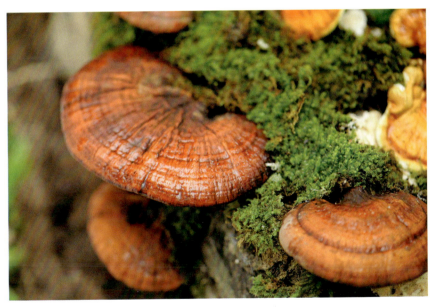

Wild Reishi Mushrooms

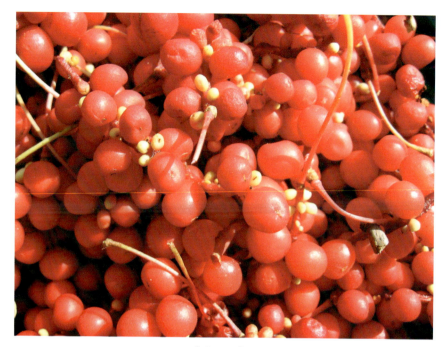

Schizandra

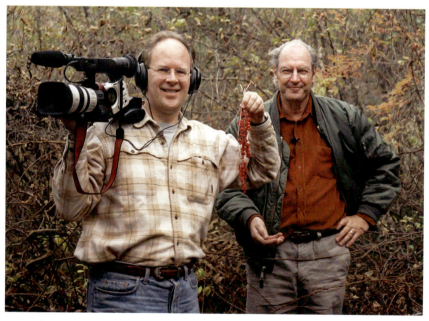

Ganga and Ron collecting Wild Schizandra on Changbai Mountain

2. SCHIZANDRA BERRIES

Schizandra Chinensis Fructus, Wu Wei Zi

"The Quintessential Herb"

Nourishes All Three Treasures: Jing, Chi, and Shen
Organ Meridians: Heart, Kidneys, Liver, Lungs,
Spiritual Qualities: Vigor, Alertness, Inner Power, Calmness, Concentration and Memory, Beauty, Psychic Power, Peacefulness

Just imagine the most pristine landscape of forests, lakes, and waterfalls on a remote ancient volcanic mountain, Changbai Shan, and you've found the best wild Schizandra in the world. Mother Nature's herbal garden of ancient China's royalty is still the ultimate source of Schizandra, the premier tonic herb for women's beauty since the ancient times of Empresses and Women of the Royal Courts of Asia. Schizandra is truly a supertonic herb of amazing capabilities.

There is an ancient Chinese legend regarding Schizandra that tells of a gentleman named Huai Nana Gong. After taking Schizandra faithfully for sixteen years, Huai had the flawless radiant complexion of a beautiful young girl, a "Jade" girl. But not only that, the strength and vitality of his skin and body could not be harmed due to the elements. The story says that he would stay dry in water and unburned in fire. But the story of Schizandra's tonifying power only starts here.

It is said that Daoist hermits savored this herbal elixir for thousands of years on their path to immortality. No matter what spiritual path you are on, this is an herb that can assist you in a multitude of ways. Known as the "Quintessential Herb," Korean tonic herbalist and Daoist Grandmaster Sung Jin Park considered these beautiful bright red berries, Schizandra, the most important and powerful herb of all Tonic Herbalism.

Why would this be? Not only does Schizandra nourish all Three Treasures: Jing, our essential primal life-giving energy; Chi, our everyday energy; and Shen, our Spirit energy, Schizandra has two other unique aspects which no other herb has been found to demonstrate.

First of all, Schizandra uniquely contains all five tastes (sour, bitter, sweet, spicy/pungent, and salty) as no other herb does. Schizandra in Chinese, Wu Wei Zi, literally means "Five Flavors Fruit." Each flavor is said to correspond to the five element energies of wood, fire, earth, metal, and water that traditional Chinese medicine states make up our human body. Each element is attracted to and nourishes one of the prime body organs. Sourness (wood element) enters the Liver, bitterness (fire element) enters the Heart, sweetness (earth element) enters the spleen, spiciness (metal element) enters the Lungs, and saltiness (water element) enters the Kidneys.

We should ideally consume all five flavors in our daily diet to maintain internal balance and proper organ nourishment. Schizandra by itself does this, nourishing and rejuvenating the Spleen, Lungs, Heart, Kidneys, and Liver.

Secondly, Schizandra opens and enters all twelve meridians of the human body, making it a total body energizer and quite possibly the most throughly tonifying herb available. These potent berries give benefit to all the functions of the body and its organs.

All these aspects of Schizandra add up to making it a powerful longevity herb, providing anti-aging capabilities for everyone, when used daily throughout one's lifetime. It does much more than just making the skin beautiful and radiant. Schizandra can be used as a Kidney tonic, as it rejuvenates the Kidneys' Jing; and a Liver tonic to cleanse, protect, nourish, and rejuvenate the Liver. A protective, safe, and effective cleansing herb, Schizandra alleviates pain, increases vision, improves hearing, is calming, and protects the adrenal glands.

Historically these vibrant dried purple berries were made into a tea or extract which became a potent Sexual tonic, powerfully rejuvenating the sexual energy of both men and women. When consumed on a regular basis, one's sexual energy noticeably increases, produces an abundance of sexual fluids, and strengthens the entire body.

This precious berry is a top blood purifier that tonifies the major functions of the mind and brain. Schizandra promotes calmness, alertness, concentration, memory, intelligence, endurance, and wisdom. It is said to also have the potential to imbue one with psychic and inner power.

Amazing Schizandra easily could be called "The Ultimate Tonic Herb" because it functions as a Yin tonic, Yang tonic, Blood tonic, Kidney tonic, Liver tonic, Mind tonic, Sex tonic, Shen Tonic, Beauty tonic, and a Longevity tonic.

Note: It is recommended that if you are making your own Schizandra tea from scratch, you soak freshly bought Schizandra berries for several hours before being using, to remove tannin. Ask the shop owner/herbalist if they have soaked the berries. When dried, the berries will look purple. If the dried berries are dark black or brown, are highly shriveled, or have many white spots on them, they are likely too old to use.

Contraindications: None.

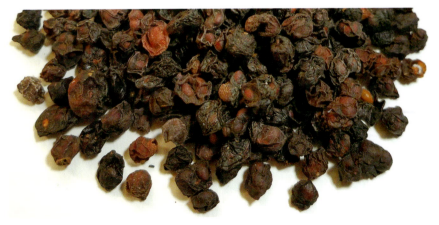

Dried Schizandra Berries

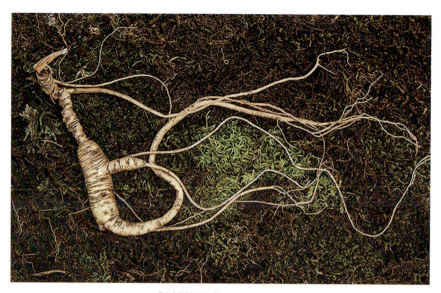

Old Wild Ginseng Root

"The root of ginseng vitalizes the five organs, calms the nerves, stops palpitations due to fright, brightens vision, improves one's intellect, removes "evil energy" (pathogenic factors), and with prolonged use, prolongs life by slowing aging and making one feel young."
– Shennong

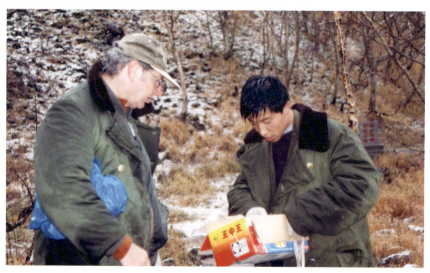

Ron buying Wild Ginseng from a collector on Changbai Mountain

3. GINSENG

Panax Ginseng, Ren Shen

"The King of Herbs"
"The Quintessential Adaptogen"

Nourishes All Three Treasures: Jing Primary, Chi, and Shen
Organ Meridians: Spleen and Lungs
Spiritual Qualities: Calmness, Harmony through Balancing, Energizing, Stimulating, Mental and Physical Strength, Elevating

The precious Ginseng root has been used in Asia for thousands of years. It is the one Asian herb that Westerners have heard of more than any other. Asian Ginseng's biological name is Panax Ginseng. The first actual record of Ginseng was found in Osagoo, Korea in 2137 BCE. The actual word "Ginseng" was discovered carved in bone and on tortoise shells used for early medicinal recordings.

This powerful herb can be found growing wild in the high mountains of Manchuria, Korea, China, and Siberia. The older in age the root is, the more powerful and more valuable the Ginseng is considered. Wild Ginseng is now a rare gem, as it is predominantly cultivated in modern times.

Most prized in ancient China by the Emperors and sages alike, the Emperor's Ginseng gardens were high on Changbai Shan, the volcanic mountain in a province of China bordering North Korea. With a history of over 5,000 years, Chinese medicine traditionally considers Ginseng the "King of Herbs" because it was used as a remedy for almost any disease.

Herbalist Doctor Li Shizhen who lived from 1518–1593 praised this herb, saying,

"Ginseng strengthens the five parts of the intestinal tract. Taking it over

a long period of time calms and strengthens the nervous system, awakens the mind, calms anxiety, makes the breath fresh, strengthens the heart, improves wisdom, and increases longevity."

Ginseng root has proven to be one of the most powerful adaptogens, which improves the body's ability to cope with physical, emotional, and environmental stress. It is uniquely both Yin and Yang, both calming and stimulating. Much current research has shown that its adaptogenic power can improve the overall functioning of individuals.

This potent root functions in a double-direction manner, bringing homeostasis to the systems of the human body. It regulates both the Central Nervous System and the Endocrine System. It helps to tonify the Kidneys in such a way as to protect the body during times of stress.

Ginseng has tested effective in lowering blood glucose and maintaining normal blood sugar levels, even for several weeks after discontinuing use. However, Asian Ginseng cannot alone prevent or treat diabetes.

Regarding blood pressure, Ginseng has the ability to regulate and restore blood pressure to normal levels in hypotense and hypertense patients.

Ginseng has a powerful influence on the Pituitary-Adrenal System. Often used as a Sex tonic, human clinical studies prove it is effective in treating impotence and some types of infertility.

Because of its influence on the metabolic system, it is found to have an anti-fatigue effects and enhance endurance, if consumed prior to exertion.

It is highly recommended for the aging due to its effect on the Nervous System. Ginseng root can improve alertness, quicken thinking, improve memory and responsiveness, reasoning ability, focus, and concentration. Chinese High School and College students are known to chew the root daily when preparing for and taking examinations.

This beautiful root has an amazing ability to rejuvenate and balance the body systems. It actually even looks like a the body of a human. Its Chinese name combines both the word for Man and Spirit, "Ren Shen." It is usually divided into three grades: Heaven, Earth, and Man, with Heaven being the best and most expensive.

Red Ginseng is mainly cultivated or semi-wild in China, North Korea, and South Korea. North Korean premium Red Ginseng is considered by many connoisseurs of ginseng to be the finest cultivated Ginseng in the world. This Ginseng is very tasty, very very yang, and produces a hot energy. It is most often used to increase physical and sexual power.

Ron's favorite cultivated Ginseng is Chinese "Shih Chu" red Ginseng from Shih Chu Valley near Changbai Mountain. Shih Chu red Ginseng is powerful yet mild. Ron says it affects body and mind, lifting the spirit and sharpening the intellect. It is almost better than wild Ginseng, but you need to get the older, larger, Heaven grade roots.

White Ginseng is also beneficial and is exported from China and South Korea. It is called "white" Ginseng because although it is dried, it has not been steamed, as has "red" Ginseng. So the difference is in the preparation. Red roots in effect are more powerful, white roots are milder, more yin, and thus good for maintenance. Red Ginseng is usually made from the best roots found.

In this fast-paced age of non-stop stress and bombardment of environmental pollutants, Ginseng's ability to calm the system and give physical and mental resilience under stress conditions is renowned.

For people wanting to maintaining an active life in the world and still maintain a rich spiritual life of activities and service, and meditation, Ginseng can give invaluable strength and emotional balance.

Sages would also use Ginseng to give themselves energy while fasting and while staying mentally calm for both meditation and spiritual cultivation. It is said that Buddhist texts describe Ginseng as being able to speed up the burning of Karma.

Contraindications: Ginseng is free of toxicity when used moderately and appropriately; it has no negative side effects. Excessive consumption may cause headaches or muscle tension for people with a yang or hot constitution, thus should be used with caution and moderation. Ginseng should never to be used by anyone experiencing an acute fever or sore throat.

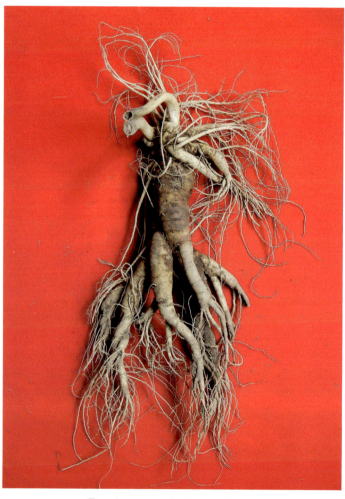

Development of Ginseng Roots

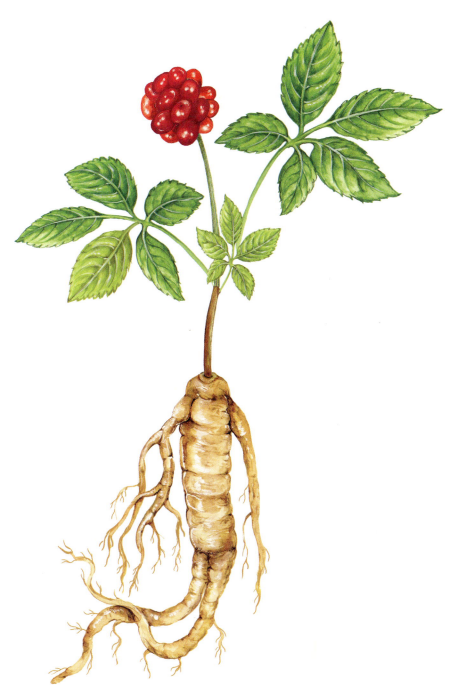
Ginseng Plant

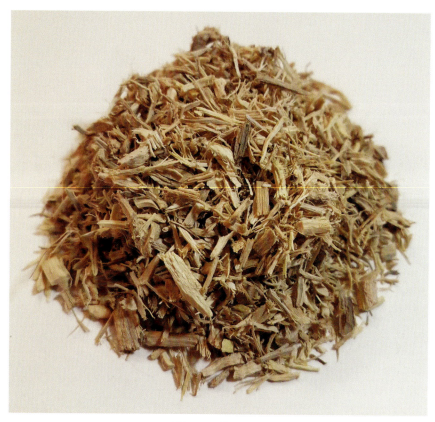
Siberian Ginseng

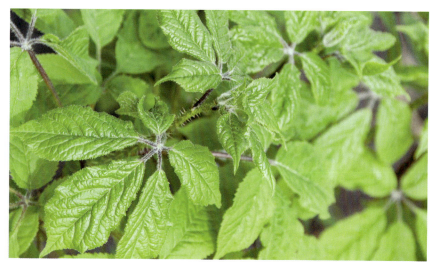
Siberian Ginseng Plant

4. SIBERIAN GINSENG

Eleutherococcus Senticosus, Ci Wu Ja

Nourishes: Jing and Chi
Organ Meridians: Spleen, Lungs, Heart, Kidneys, and Liver
Spiritual Qualities: Strength, Endurance, Energy, Alertness, Calmness, Expansion of Abilities

Eleutherococcos is a powerful adaptogenic root used in tonic herbalism for centuries. It is commonly called Siberian Ginseng. It is a relative of the true ginseng, Panax Ginseng, however there is no physical resemblance to it. Wild Siberian Ginseng is indigenous to Siberia, Mongolia, and Northeastern China. A popular herb of Martial artists. It is used as a Stimulant Tonic that can increase immediate energy and longterm energy.

As a famous adaptogenic herb used around the world, it aids one in building and enhancing strength in any athletic endeavor, physical labor, or outdoor work and is especially helpful in cold environments.

Currently it is useful, as well, for handling stressful and demanding careers. It can assist one in both expanding work capacity and raising the quality of work to another level. As a mild stimulant, it can immediately increase the work capacity of an individual. It can improve alertness, auditory acuity, visual acuity, and night vision. It is also known to calm the nerves, which is always useful in stressful environments.

For centuries it has been used to increase physical and mental endurance, to build blood, and to improve memory. It strengthens those recovering from extreme exercise, overexertion physically and mentally, surgery, and illness. It is now widely used to regulate blood sugar levels and is especially good for athletes in training and competitions.

Siberian Ginseng improves the ability of the human body to absorb and efficiently use oxygen. It is beneficial for athletes requiring respiratory endurance, such as mountain climbers at high altitudes, long distance racers, triathlon athletes, and competitive performers. It has been used to prevent altitude sickness. It has even proven beneficial for Russian cosmonauts in space travel.

A powerful Chi tonic, it invigorates the functions of the Spleen, Kidney, and Liver. Eleutherococcus offers relief from the pain of rheumatic arthritis, regulates blood sugar in the treatment of diabetes, and regulates and normalizes blood pressure. As an immune modulator, it builds resistance to infectious and chronic diseases.

You will only find the finished product in shops if you live in America. A very precious commodity, it takes fifty pounds of the raw Siberian Ginseng root to produce one pound of extract.

Contraindications: None. A very safe herb. Perhaps the healthiest and safest stimulant known to man.

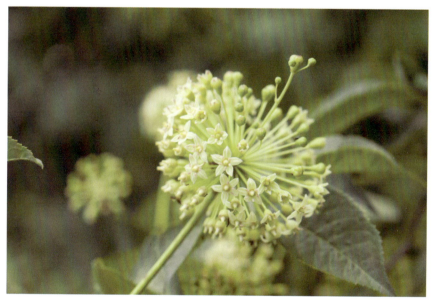

Siberian Ginseng Flower

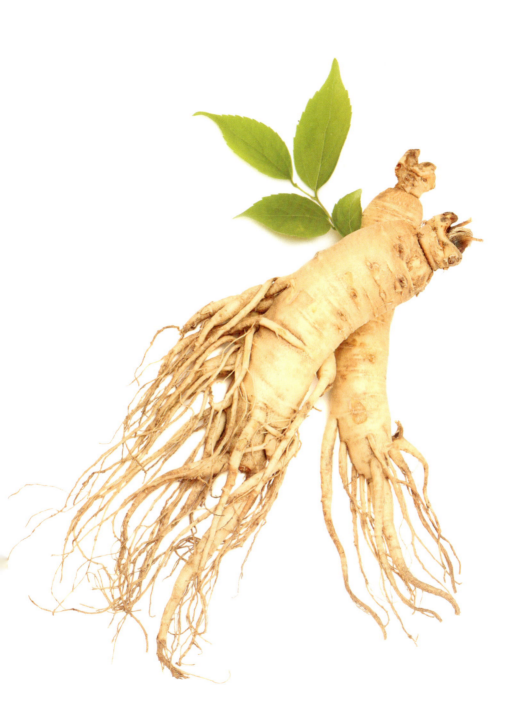

Siberian Ginseng Roots

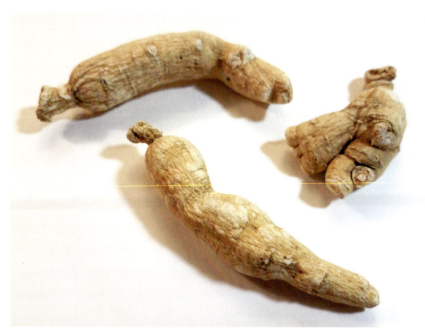

American Ginseng Roots

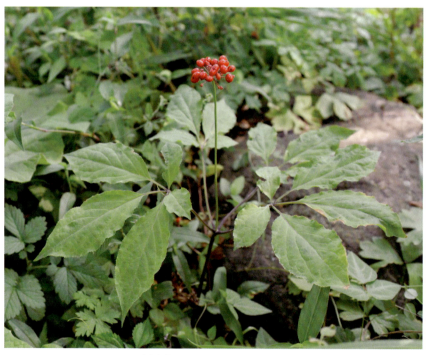

Wild American Ginseng Plant

5. AMERICAN GINSENG

Panax Quinquefolius L
Xi Yang Shen, Hua Qi Shen

Nourishes: Yin and Chi
Organ Meridians: Lungs, Spleen, and Stomach
Spiritual Qualities: Energy, Endurance, and Heightened Alertness

American Ginseng is a Yin and Chi tonic and is highly respected by Asians. Different than Asian Ginseng, American Ginseng is good for people with a warmer or hot constitution or those living in a hot climate, because it is naturally cooling and mild. It is an adaptogenic herb that gives one energy, endurance, and heightened alertness. It heightens alertness, but it is not a stimulant as is Panax Ginseng. It has been found to be significantly strengthening for new mothers.

Generally the types of constitution this would be useful for are individuals who tend to have at least one of the following: lots of energy, a high metabolism, tend to be aggressive, have a ruddy complexion, or have high blood pressure.

It is excellent for nourishing the lungs, skin, and stomach. Chinese often use it for dry coughs from smog, smoking, or other causes because it can moisten and cool the lungs.

Not surprisingly, American Ginseng roots and leaves were traditionally used for medicinal purposes by Native Americans.

Wild American Ginseng is the best, but is now extremely rare to find. A premium find would be a twenty-pound wild root. It is now mainly cultivated. The largest percentage of American Ginseng is cultivated in Wisconsin, USA and Ontario, Canada.

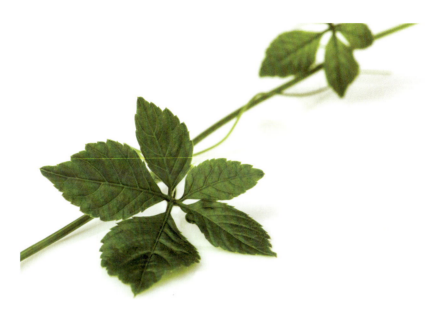

Gynostemma – Five Leaf Herb

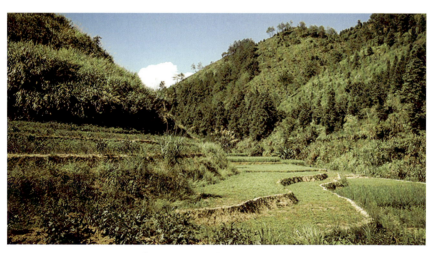

Gynostemma fields in China

6. GYNOSTEMMA

Gynostemma Pentaphyllum, Jiao Gu Lan

"The Magical Grass"

Nourishes All Three Treasures: Jing, Chi and Shen
Organ Meridians: Spleen, Lungs, Kidneys, Liver and Heart
Spiritual Qualities: Balance, Calmness, Alertness, Longevity

Gynostemma's reputation as a super anti-aging herb has had a long reign in Asia. It is among only a handful of Supertonic Herbs that nourish all Three Treasures. Today it has become one of the most popular Tonic Herbs in Asia.

So beautiful to look out over the deep green fields of Gynostemma, the magical grass is renowned for enhancing longevity. Wild Gynostemma grown in pristine mountain forests and fields is the most prized, as it is highly potent, and rare. Its most superior environment is Southeastern China.

Interestingly, the mountainous region of Guizhou is famous for its high number of centenarians who researchers found had one thing in common, drinking Gynostemma tea. The centenarians studied also had very low occurrences of Alzheimer's disease, cancer, diabetes, and high blood pressure. Gynostemma is also indigenous to South Korea and North Vietnam. Today it is cultivated in Japan and Thailand, as well as China and other parts of Asia, and has gained a sweeter taste.

Called "Jiao Gu Lan" in the Chinese language, this herb is a major broad spectrum adaptogenic herb, validated for its longevity power. As a super adaptogen it has double-directional activity in many functional systems of the body. Through continuous consumption, Gynostemma is able to generate a protective quality, strengthening a person on many levels, including the immune system. It both supports and helps to maintain normal healthy immune functions. The real power here is that it can regulate systems of the body, bringing them back into balance or homeostasis. Since ancient times, it has been used as a cure-all herb in Chinese Medicine. Gynostemma as a tea or elixir is well-worth drinking on a daily basis by people of any age. This magical green grass is also able to strengthen the mind, calm the nerves, and reduce oxygen deficiency at high altitudes. It can create a perfect balance for meditators and spiritual practitioners cultivating wisdom, who need to stay mentally and emotionally calm, yet alert. Gynostemma's regulating ability is calming to someone overexcited, yet stimulating when they are feeling sluggish or lethargic.

While it is a treatment for elders to slow down aging and prevent feebleness and senility, in China, the young and athletic also use it to increase vigor and reduce fatigue. It has been called the Southern Ginseng by the Chinese.

Gynostemma's therapeutic qualities have been successful in lowering high blood pressure and lowering cholesterol, strengthening the immune system, building anti-inflammatory response, fighting colds, protecting the liver, improving digestion, reducing mucus in chronic bronchitis, and inhibiting tumors in cancer patients. Researchers from Japan find its effective assistance in a vast array of disease including cardiovascular disease and diabetes. A 2012 German study by the Institute of Biochemistry discovered something very promising about Gynostemma extract. Brain tissue treated with Gynostemma extract 48 hours before ischemia were protected from further injury. Ischemia is a brain injury caused from loss of blood flow to the brain causing a stroke. (Phytomedicine, Volume 19. Issue 8-9, June 15, 2012)

Considered by some as the "Weight Loss Herb," with the same regulating functionality it can assist in increasing metabolism, losing weight, and balancing blood sugar. Athletes who consume Gynostemma are able to build more lean muscle mass than those who do not.

Contraindications: Nontoxic and safe for consumption.

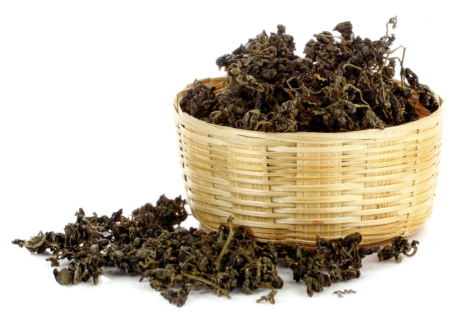

Dried Gynostemma

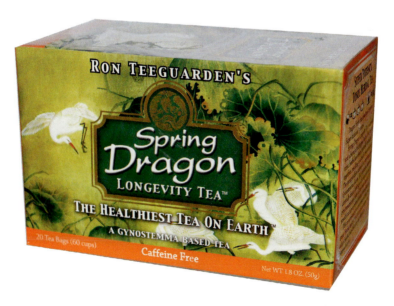

Spring Dragon Longevity Tea is my favorite tea, and I try to drink it every day.
The base is Gynostemma, known as "Magical Grass" in China, along with
Schizandra, Lycium, Astragalus, Siberian Ginseng, and Luo Han Guo.
I believe that Spring Dragon Longevity Tea is the healthiest tea in the world.

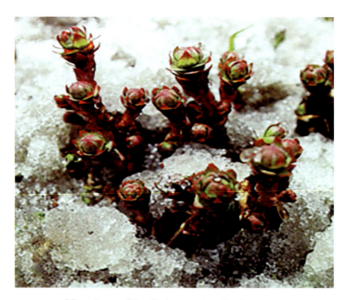

Himalayan Rhodiola growing in the snow

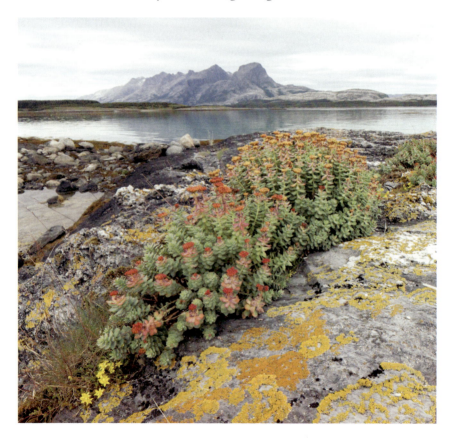

7. RHODIOLA

Rhodiola Sacra, Tibetan Rhodiola, Hong Jing Tian, Rhodiola Rosea, Golden Root

Nourishes: Jing, Chi, and Shen
Spiritual Qualities: Energized, Physical Endurance, Stamina, Contentment, Mental Clarity, Intelligence, Feeling of Well-being, Wisdom, Elevating Spirit

Grown wild in China and Tibet for thousand of years, Rhodiola has long been considered a sacred herb by Buddhist monks, especially those living in mountainous regions of Tibet and Bhutan. Rhodiola naturally increases oxygen in the blood, which activates pleasure centers in the brain and produces feelings of well-being, the expansion of wisdom and contentment.

Rhodiola has a rich history around the world. In China the Emperors sent expeditions to Siberia in search of the "Golden Root" for preparing medicine. This Russian Rhodiola is know as Rhodiola Rosea. Mongolian physicians treated patients with cancer or tuberculosis with Rhodiola root. In Greece in AD 77, the physician, botanist, and pharmacologist Dioscorides documented the application of the herb in his classic medical text, *De Materia Medica*. In Scandinavia, Vikings used the energizing herb to increase their physical power, strength, and endurance.

Himalayan Rhodiola, "Rhodiola Sacra," grows wild in a harsh environment of extreme high altitude, cold, snow, and ice. It is a rare gem to find but believed to be the most potent variety of this herb, which has yet to be cultivated in such an environment.

The benefits of Rhodiola are valuable for everyone. Rhodiola is a remarkable herb said to function as a potent adaptogen that stabilizes and normalizes the bodies functions. Its impact is truly extensive: it strengthens the nervous system, fights depression, enhances immunity, increases stamina—elevating the capacity for exercise, enhances memory, weight reduction, increases sexual function, increases energy levels, enhances work performance, eliminates fatigue, and prevents high altitude sickness.

Beyond mental well-being, Rhodiola also has the ability to improve overall brain functioning. Studies have demonstrated that Rhodiola extract enhances memorization and the ability to concentrate over prolonged periods. It can even be used as a successful prescription for depression, schizophrenia, emotional instability, and anxiety. It stimulates brain receptivity to the neurotransmitters, serotonin and dopamine, which are known to increase cognitive function. Athletes and those wanting to lose weight will find Rhodiola helpful, as it has been shown to shorten recovery time after prolonged workouts and to improve sleep patterns. Rosavin, an active compound found in Rhodiola, has been proven to assist the body of those losing weight when calories are restricted.

Scientists studying the heart have found that Rhodiola can decrease the risk of heart disease by decreasing the harmful blood lipids. It regulates the heartbeat and counteracts heart arrhythmias.

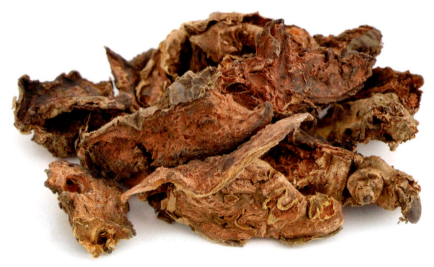

Wild Tibetan Rhodiola Roots

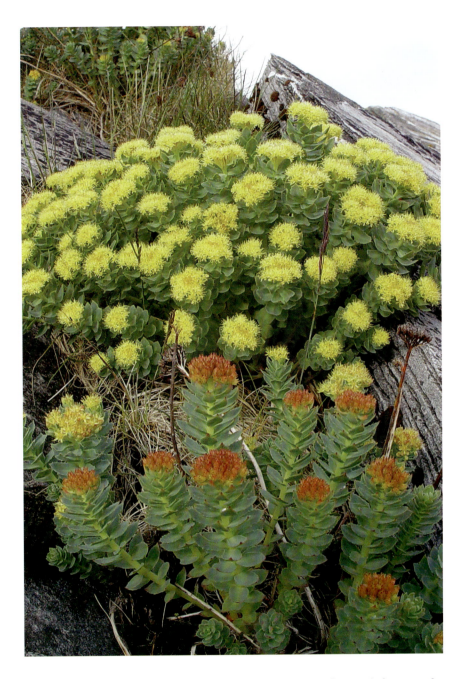

Rhodiola grows in China, Tibet, the Himalayas, Central Asia, and cold regions, including much of the Arctic, Russia, Eastern North America, parts of Northern Europe, Iceland, and sea cliffs and mountains at altitudes of up to 7500 feet.

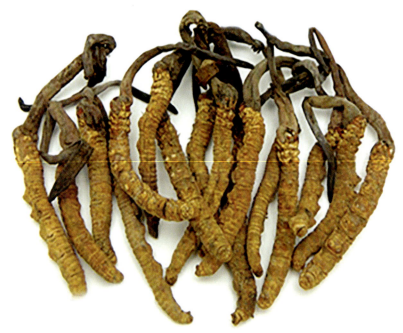

Cordyceps

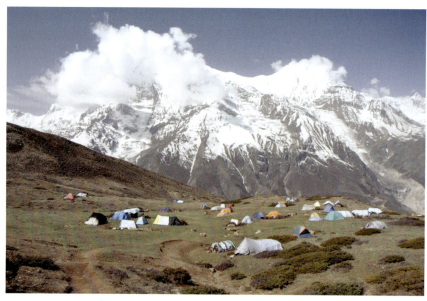

Cordyceps harvesting camp in the Himalayas

8. CORDYCEPS

Cordyceps Sinensis, Dong Chong Xia Cao

Nourishes: Yin Jing, Yang Jing, and Chi
Organ Meridians: Kidneys and Lungs
Spiritual Qualities: Strength, Rejuvenation, Youthfulness, Vigor, Longevity

One of the most highly prized treasures of Tonic Herbalism in the world is the unusual substance known as Cordyceps. Cordyceps is one of the three herbal gems of the Himalayas, which also includes Snow Lotus and Rhodiola. It is one of the main substances used by Asians for rejuvenation on a deep level. It replenishes our essential Yin Jing, as well as, Yang Jing.

Cordyceps are unusual in that they are actually mushrooms that grow on the heads of caterpillars. The caterpillars become their fertilizer, so to speak. The result is a 100% vegetarian fungi that actually resembles the shape of the caterpillar.

Proven beneficial through practical application for centuries, and modern research, Cordyceps are used throughout Asia, especially China and Japan. They are used primarily to strengthen Kidney essence, Yang Jing, and Yin Jing energy. This affects sexual functions, mind power, healing capacity, and structural integrity of the body.

As a Sex tonic it is top-notch if used continuously over a long period of time. It can also treat frigidity, impotence, and infertility. Structurally it strengthens the skeletal system, lower back, ankles and knees. It is also a great tonic for people recovering from injury, illness, surgery, or after giving birth.

A major immune system strengthener, it assists in building resistance to a wide range of bacteria, fungi, and viruses, and prevents various diseases. Research has shown that it has strong anti-tumor activity. That not being impressive enough, it is beneficial to the cardiovascular system, as it helps regulate blood pressure and strengthens the heart muscle.

Cordyceps are an excellent Lung tonic for those with weak lungs suffering from wheezing, shortness of breath, or chronic coughing. Or just to increase respiratory power for outdoor labor, sports, and athletic performance. It is also considered an Athlete's tonic for building muscles. It is a favorite herb of Martial Artists.

Wild Cordyceps are extremely rare; and if found, quite expensive, as they grow in high mountains regions. They are very dangerous to hunt for, as they are often on the edge of steep cliffs in the Himalayas in Tibet, Mongolia, or high peaks in China. Each year many harvesters are injured by falling off cliffs. This unique herbal substance can also be found in India and Nepal.

Himalayan Cordyceps are the premium choice of herbal connoisseurs. High quality Cordyceps are large in size and light brown in color. Wild Cordyceps are the most potent and beneficial. Yet today in Chinese herbal stores, you will usually find cultivated Cordyceps developed through a new fermentation process devoid of caterpillar, but which still makes a premium tonic elixir.

Contraindications: Safe. Not to be used when experiencing a fever.

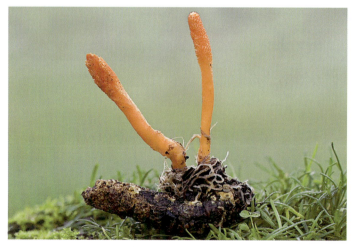

Cordyceps (photo by Jose Ramon Pato)

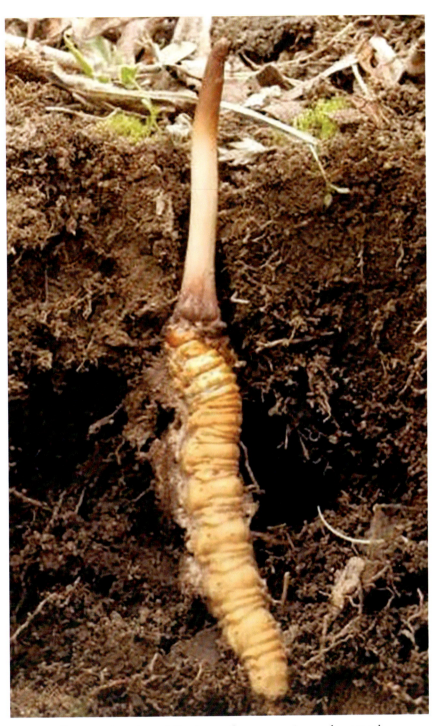
Cross section view of Cordyceps fungus growing underground

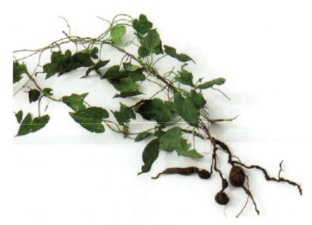

He Shou Wu

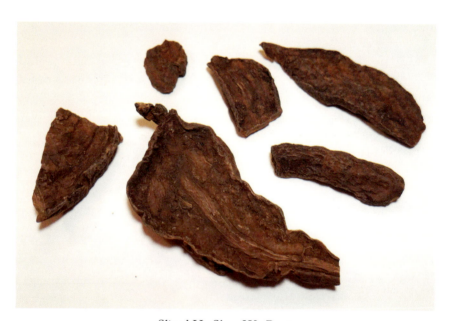

Sliced He Shou Wu Root

9. POLYGONUM

Polygonum Multiflorum, Polygonaceae Shou Wu, He Shou Wu,

Nourishes: Yin Jing and Blood
Organ Meridians: Liver and Kidneys
Spiritual Qualities: Energizing, Calming, Strength, Youthfulness, Longevity

He Shou Wu stands out in Tonic herbalism as the primary Jing tonic. Its biological name is Polygonum Multiflorum. The first found record of He Shou Wu is from the Qin Dynasty, 221-206 BCE, written by the herbalist An Qi. Qi was said to be a specialist in miraculous herbs.

Polygonum is a fundamental aid in the practice of the Daoist inner arts. Both Daoist Master Sung Jin Park and his Master, Moo San Do Sha, recommended that this tonic be taken every day, as it has the power to build and preserve your primal essence-Jing. It accomplishes this by supporting the Liver and Kidneys, making it one of the most important and powerful anti-aging herbs in Tonic Herbalism. Its only match is the Lycium fruit.

He Shou Wu, made from the tuberous root, is a great strengthener of the human body. It is renowned for maintaining the strength and stability of the lower back and knees through tonifying two of our vital organs, the Liver and the Kidneys. In response, they nourish the blood which fortifies the bones, muscles, tendons, and ligaments. It also improves the function of the adrenal glands and aids in clearing the eyes and improving vision. It also performs as an effective Blood tonic, cleaning the blood and strengthening red blood cell membranes, while promoting cell growth and development. A favorite of athletes and martial artists for all the above reasons, and for providing resilience and stamina. It is undoubtedly one of the most powerful longevity promoting herbs available.

Yet it is probably most famous in Asia, as they believe it has the capacity to return gray hair back to its natural black or adult color, giving the look of youthfulness. The herbal plant Polygonum Multiflorum grows in the mountains of central and southern China. It was named He Shou Wu by the Chinese, after the man who discovered it. What is consumed is the tubular root, which must be prepared first, not taken raw, in order to be used as a regularly-consumed tonic herb. It is uniquely energizing to the body and calming to the nerves.

Considered the primary Sex tonic to enhance the fertility of both women and men, He Shou Wu builds and preserves your primal essence—your functional reserve—and increases the sperm and vitalizes the ova. When planning to conceive a child, both parents should consume the tonic.

Caution: Raw unprepared He Shou Wu functions as a laxative and should not be consumed on a long-term basis. Prepared He Shou Wu functions as a tonic herb and can be taken on a regular basis.

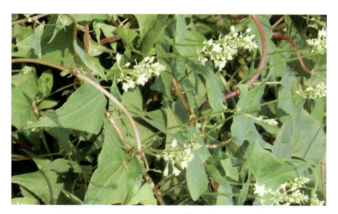

Polygonum Multiform (He Shou Wu)

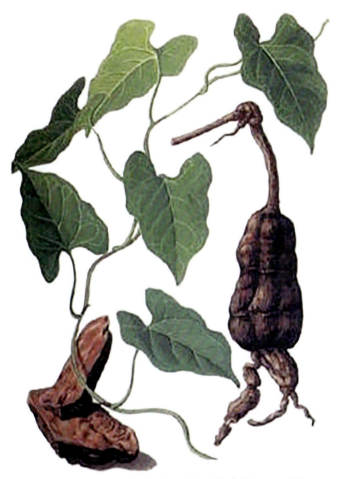

Polygonum Multiform (He Shou Wu) Plant and Root

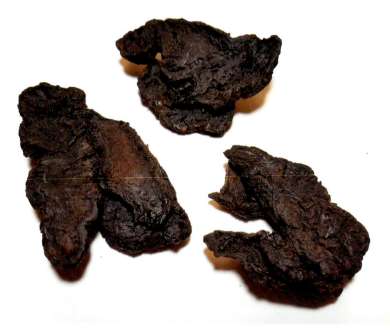

Prepared Rehmannia

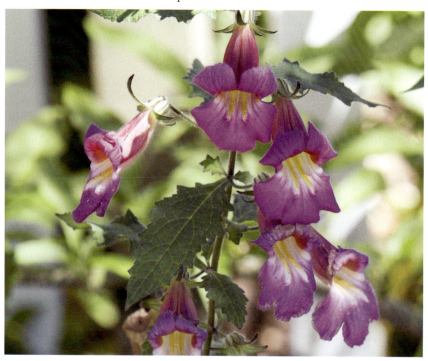

Rehmannia Flowers

10. REHMANNIA ROOT

Rehmannia Glutinosa, *Chinese Foxglove*
Di Huang

"The Kidneys' Own Food"

Nourishes: Yin Jing and Blood
Organ Meridians: Kidneys, Liver, and Heart
Spiritual Qualities: Rejuvenation, Longevity

A primary Longevity herb since ancient times, Rehmannia has been said to be "the Kidneys' own food." This powerful root must be prepared first through steaming to access supertonic benefits for our primal life-giving organs: the Kidneys, Liver, and Heart. Combining the steamed Rehmannia with other Chi tonics improves its assimilation into the body. After being prepared the root will take on a black color.

Benefiting both men and women, prepared Rehmannia is a potent Yin Jing tonic that quickly provides effective nourishment to our Kidneys. Acting as a Sex tonic, it strengthens the reproductive functions of the body, thus enhancing fertility when also combined with other similarly benefiting Tonic Herbs.

Rehmannia is a significant herb for women. It functions as a blood building tonic for the female body, and its warming nature is beneficial to the uterus. Prepared Rehmannia can prevent painful menstruation in addition to enhancing fertility.

High quality prepared Rehmannia has a soft, fine texture that can be easily chewed and tastes very sweet.

Contraindications: Use with caution if you have a weak digestive system that is prone to diarrhea; it should be combined with other Chi tonics, such as Polygonum, to avoid such issue.

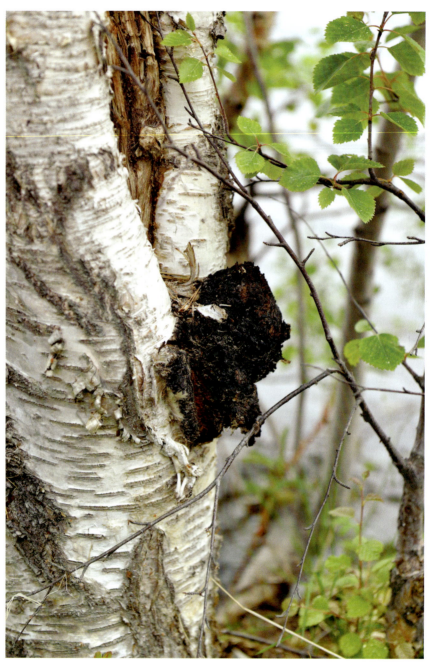

Chaga growing on a birch tree

11. CHAGA

Inonotus Obliquus, Bai Hua Rong

"A Gift from God"
"A Precious Gift of Nature"

Nourishes: Jing, Chi, and Shen
Organ Meridians: Kidneys, Liver, Lungs, and Spleen
Spiritual Qualities: Rejuvenative, Protecting, Radiant Health, Youthfulness, Longevity

Russia's best kept secret is the highly acclaimed supertonic Chaga Mushroom, found growing wild in subarctic old birch forests, a cold, harsh climate where the temperature drops to 40 below zero. Chaga is a parasitic fungus that gains it highest medicinal value when specifically grown on birch trees and harvested only after reaching its full maturity at twenty years. Following the Di Dao philosophy, the best Chaga in the world is said to come from these remote Siberian birch forests.

Chaga, the black tree fungus, often referred to as "A Gift from God," was famed in Russian herbalism and Siberian folk medicine for hundreds or even thousands of years, for possessing the ability to help humans adapt to cold, harsh climates by boosting the immune system. Folk medicine used Chaga as a tea, and it was often used to treat gastritis and other related gastrointestinal problems.

Yet, it is said that it took Noble Prize Laureate and novelist Aleksandr Solzhenitsyn to awaken the West to this amazing Fungi. In 1968 Solzhenitsyn published his book *The Cancer Ward*, in which he describes "the tea from the birch tree mushroom," its healing components, and its potential benefits to cancer patients.

The most research on Chaga has been done in Russia and Scandinavia, where according to Christopher Hobbs, extracts of chaga were approved as an anticancer drug, called Befungin, in Russia as early as 1955 and has been reported successful in treating breast, lung, cervical, and stomach cancers. Befungin is still used today.

More research is needed in the Western countries to determine Chaga's full potential for various cancers and other degenerative diseases. However, similar to other medicinal mushrooms, Chaga, like Reishi, can be used as a supportive adjunct to chemo and radiation therapies. Betulin in Chaga is known to help detoxify the Liver and protect against the potentially damaging effects of radiation or chemotherapy chemicals. High amounts of antioxidants in Chaga, including melanin (that binds to radioactive isotopes), are specifically helpful for rejuvenating healthy immune responses. For ages, Chinese and Asian herbalists have highly regarded Chaga as a longevity herb, preserving youthfulness and radiant health. A traditional superior herb, acknowledged by the ancient Chinese herbalist Shennong in the first printed herbal compendium, *Shennong Bencao Jing (Herbal Classic of Shennong)*, he described it as "The King of Herbs" and "A Precious Gift of Nature." It is commonly categorized as a high quality Chi tonic; it is also used as a Shen tonic, as well as an outstanding Kidney tonic and cleanser, and Liver tonic. It is said that the Chinese frequently use an extract of Chaga to thoroughly detox the Liver, Lungs, and Spleen, cleanse the bowels, and prevent Kidney stones.

More modern interest in the positive benefits of Chaga and its biological components have spurred research by the Chinese and other Asian research communities, leaving its extensive potential wide open. Why so much interest? Studies of the biochemical components of Chaga exhibit a wide variety of biological functions, including anti-bacterial, anti-allergic, anti-inflammatory, anti-viral, anti-oxidative, anti-inflammatory, anti-tumor, cytotoxic, anti-platelet aggregation, anti-diabetic, anti-dementia and anti-viral activity. Chaga's melanin shows strong DNA/gene protective effects (genoprotective) including protection of DNA damage from oxidative stress.

To highlight a few of these strong supported benefits, Siberian Chaga has been proven to be a very powerful antioxidant. Studies from Tufts University have found it to be an even more potent free radical scavenger (scoring the highest ORAC) than any natural food, including the most popular dietary antioxidants you are familiar with, including blueberries, goji berries, and acai berries.

Best of all, Inonotus Obliquus is a superb immune builder and fighter. Chaga is well-known as a powerful double-direction adaptogen having an unrivaled immune response. Undoubtedly a significant superfood for autoimmune disorders. A great protector of health overall, Chaga is a superb immune modulating tonic—strengthening, balancing, supporting, regulating, and maintaining body functioning at its optimal homeostasis.

Chaga can be found growing wild in many colder regions around the world beyond Siberian Russia. This includes Korea, China, Northern Europe, Canada, Northern America, and Scandinavia.

Contraindications: None known. Chaga is very safe and free from side effects. Chaga may be consumed as a tonic herb over a long period of time (indefinitely) in moderate amounts. Avoid using if you are on blood thinning drugs or medication to lower blood sugar (Chaga may also lower blood sugar).

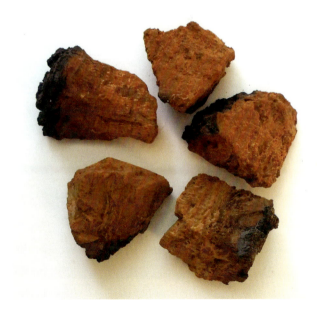

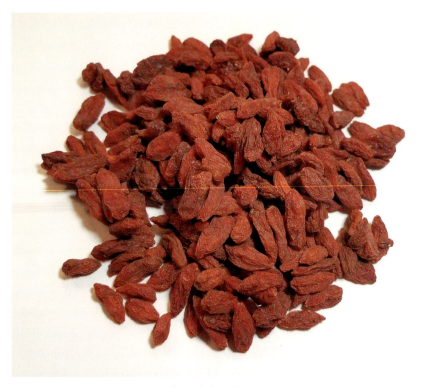

Dried Goji Berries

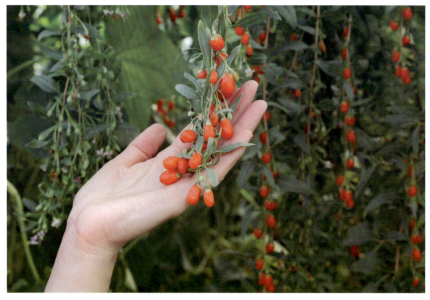

Wild Lycium—Goji Berries

12. LYCIUM FRUIT

Lycium Barbarum L,
Goji Berries,
Gou Qi Zi,
Chinese Wolfberries

"The Happiness Herb"

Nourishes: Yin Jing and Blood
Organ Meridians: Liver, Kidneys, Lungs
Spiritual Qualities: Happiness, Cheerfulness, Strength, Vitality, Longevity

The sweet-tasting red Lycium fruit is widely known as the Goji Berry. Prolonged consumption of these delicious berries promotes cheerfulness and vitality. In the West, children learn that to eat an apple a day keeps the doctor away. In China, it is traditionally said that eating a handful of Goji Berries will make you happy the entire day. And if you consume them long enough, you won't be able to stop smiling!

Many well-known Daoists and Herbalists who attained great longevity and wisdom have revered Lycium as a herb of longevity. Nutritious and potent, Lycium tonifies the Kidneys and Liver, and builds Jing. It balances Yin and Yang. It makes an excellent Yin Jing, Yang Jing tonic and Blood tonic.

Two master herbalists of the sixth and seventh century A.D., Tao Hong-Jing and Sun Si-Miao, were proponents of longevity during a time in which the life expectancy was only 27 years. Both were known to consume Goji daily. Tao Hong-Jing lived to be 80 years old. Chinese Herbalist Sun Si-Miao, who was considered an expert in Longevity, wrote two famous books that are essentially compendiums of China's medical achievements from known history up until the seventh century. Sun was born with a very weak constitution and was a sickly child. He quickly took to the study of herbalism to improve his health, later devoting his entire life to the practice and study of medicine. Sun Si-Miao is said to have eaten Goji berries morning and evening his entire life and completed his last book a year before he died, at 101. This is why Goji Berries have developed a reputation for giving one a long, vigorous, and happy life.

Asian athletes and martial artists have prized Goji, as it has the ability to strengthen the legs and increase vitality. It has also proven successful in fighting obesity. In fact, research found that drinking Goji morning and afternoon as a tea helped patients significantly lose weight.

Goji is a potent tonic for vision. When consumed continuously it is said to maintain healthy vision, brighten the eyes, and improve vision.

For centuries Goji Berries have been grown and picked on Heaven Mountain (Changbai Shan), as it is the Di Dao, the most perfect native environment for this species. The Goji Berries from this province are often called Xin Jiang Goji. Xin Jiang Province has the longest duration of daylight of all the provinces in China and Tibet. So these berries are grown drenched and nurtured in 2500 to 3300 hours of sunlight per year!

Goji Berries support our health in many ways. They possess powerful immune-supporting phytochemicals which when mixed with other specific herbs protect our nervous system, strengthen the Kidneys, Liver, Lungs, and the Heart and the entire cardiovascular system. They are a great mood enhancer.

This delicious superfood berry contains an abundance of health-promoting nutrients: high amounts of vitamin C and beta carotene (the vitamin A precursor), vitamins B1, B2, B6, E, and more than twenty trace minerals, including calcium, organic germanium, selenium, zinc, copper, phosphorus, and iron, plus 18 amino acids, 6 essential fatty acids, polysaccharides, and an abundance of zeaxanthin. It is also considered an alkaline food.

Lycium Berries enhance normal sexual functioning and when mixed with other yang herbs make a great sex tonic, enhancing sexual fluids and fertility. In China, it is used by pregnant mothers in the first trimester to prevent morning sickness.

Contraindications: Lycium is not toxic, but it should not be used in the case of a fever caused by infection or if you suffer from a Spleen deficiency with diarrhea. If you are on blood pressure medication, consult your doctor first; most likely you would need to adjust your medication if you consume the berries on a regular basis. Western convention recommends avoiding them while pregnant or breast-feeding. Goji "might" cause an allergic reaction in people who are allergic to tobacco, peaches, tomatoes, or nuts.

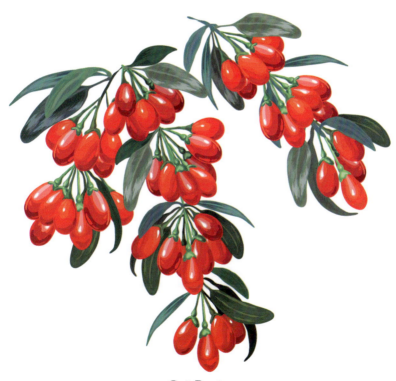

Goji Berries

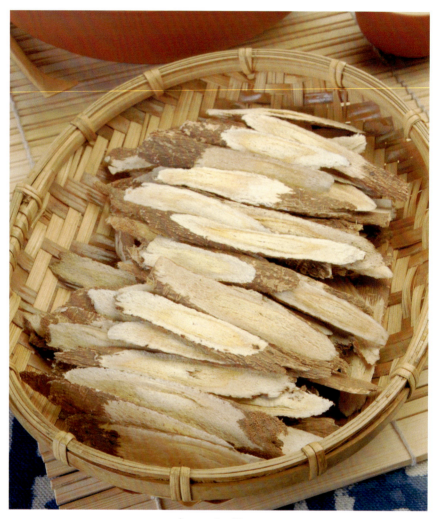
Astragalus Root

13. ASTRAGALUS

Astragalus Membranaceus, Huang Qi

"The Great Protector"

Nourishes: Chi and Blood
Organ Meridians: Spleen and Lungs
Spiritual Qualities: Energy, Endurance, Strength, Longevity

Astragalus is known as "The Great Protector," thought to be the most widely used herb across Asia for the last 2000 years until now. This powerful root is one of the most potent tonics for your health because it is a great strengthener and energizer. It fortifies the immune system, the defense field of our human body. In Asia it is a primary herb in cold-fighting formulas and Blood tonics, and is often consumed daily to strengthen the body.

The plant root is used to create a tonic extract or tea. Astragalus root helps develop protective Chi. Astragalus can generate and tonify the protective Chi that circulates over the surface layer of the body, under the skin and muscles. It produces free flow Chi. This protective energy is known as "Wei Qi" in Chinese, it is Yang energy. As an immune modulator, it tones this protective energy that runs not just under the skin layer but also penetrates into our organ systems. Internally, at a deeper level, the primary energy of the body's metabolic, respiratory, and eliminative functions are strengthened by Astragalus.

One key ability of Astragalus Root is to fortify the "Upright Chi." Upright Chi is the energy allocated by the body to maintain a healthy upright posture and to maintain the correct positioning of the organs in their natural battle with gravity. As one gets older, this upright Chi is naturally depleted and organs in the abdominal and pelvic region prolapse, meaning they drop. This herb is helpful for prolapse of organs such as the stomach, uterus, or hernia of the intestines. This strengthening herb is also beneficial in exhaustion, chronic fatigue, and wound healing. It is very useful in producing faster recovery from illness and surgery.

This sweet-tasting yellow root is slightly diuretic and detoxifying. It helps those who have slow-healing wounds, excessive sweating, loose stool, chronic diarrhea, or can't get over chronic colds. For younger people, it is often recommended to use Astragalus over Ginseng for increased energy.

The importance of Astragalus extract's immunomodulating effects has been proven by American university research to improve the immune response to those treated with radiation and chemotherapy as cancer treatments. It is approved in many other countries for a higher and faster recovery rate. This immune-modulating activity is also effective at both building immune response and suppressing excessive response in autoimmune conditions such as allergies and arthritis. Interestingly, it is also a strong tonic for bone marrow. It may be used in any tonic formula to strengthen the body.

Yogis, Meditators, Athletes, Hikers, Outdoor Workers? Astragalus specifically is used to strengthen the legs and arms, especially in the cold, because it is both strengthening and warming. Anyone who is consistently physically active could greatly benefit from using this tonic herb. It is fortifies our first defense against the elements of Nature.

Luckily, this herb is prevalent in many environments around the world, from Northern China and Mongolia to Europe, the Western USA, and Canada.

Contraindications: It should not be used in the acute phase of a flu, but during the convalescing stage. If you are prone to flatulence, use less Astragalus and add herbs like Cardamom to a tea.

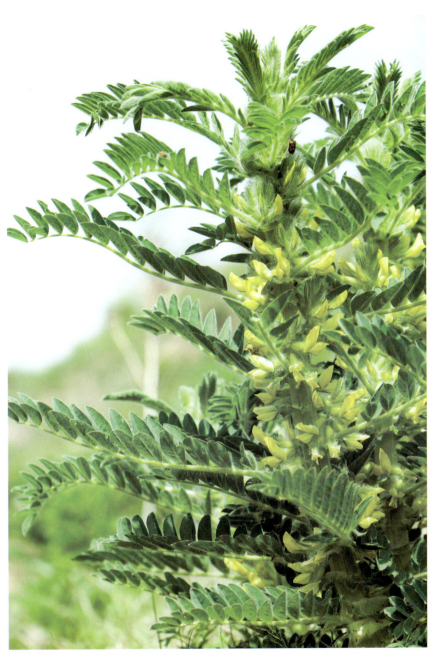
Astragalus Plant

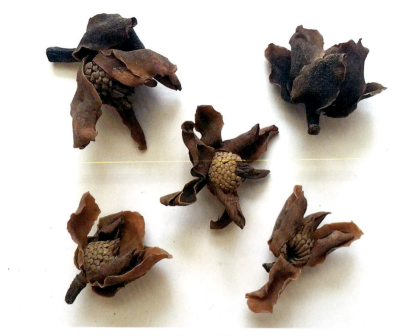

Albizzia Flowers

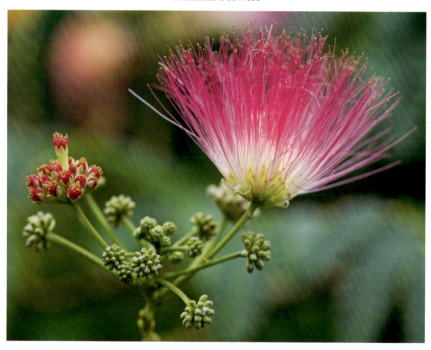

14. ALBIZZIA

*Albizia Julibrissin,
He Huan Hua (flower),
He Huan Pi (bark)*

"The Happiness Herb"

Nourishes: Shen
Organ Meridians: Heart and Liver
Spiritual Qualities: Relieving, Calming, Happiness, Emotionally Uplifting, Stabilizing, Elevating Spirit

The exotic Albizzia tree produces both flowers and bark that are famous in China for their Shen stabilizing abilities, so supporting and beneficial to Tonic Herbalism. In the West it is known as the distinctively beautiful and fragrant Mimosa Tree. Native to China, Persia, Korea, and Japan, it grows in temperate zones around the world. Albizzia herbal remedies both nourish and strengthen the Heart and the Liver. This sweet tasting herb can be used for people suffering severe depression, emotional heartache, fright, worry, upsets, and grieving great losses, by calming and lifting one's spirit.

The delicate Albizzia Flower is the ultimate Shen tonic because it has a strong mood-elevating quality. It elevates, lifts, and builds Shen, as well as stabilizing it. It is even stronger than the bark itself in elevating the mood and consciousness of the severely depressed. It can be used for heart-break and despair. Even severe conditions such as paranoia, anger, and despondency can be treated with this herb. I can't imagine any herbalist wanting to be without Albizzia; it could be an emotional lifesaver.

Albizzia Bark is also an excellent Shen stabilizer; calming chronic emotional upsets. It can improve conditions of anxiety, sleeplessness due to emotions, irritableness, anger, forgetfulness, excessive worry, and any chronic emotion.

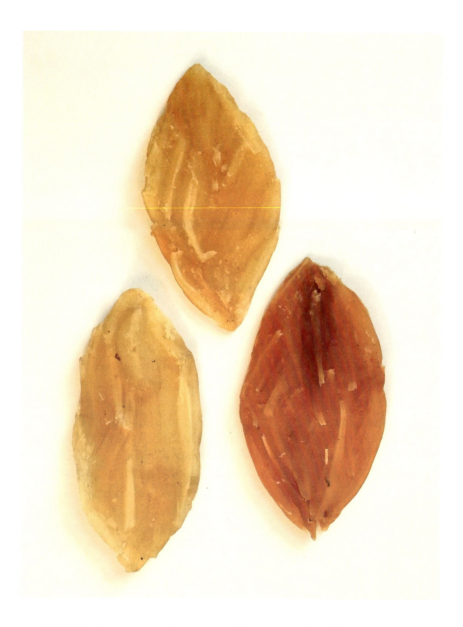

"Wild Asparagus Root is said to open the Heart Center, allowing Shen to flourish, manifesting as feelings of love, goodwill, patience, and peace of mind."

~ Ron Teeguarden
The Ancient Wisdom of the Chinese Tonic Herbs

15. WILD ASPARAGUS ROOT

Asparagus Cochinchinensis, Tian Men Dong

Nourishes All Three Treasures: Yin Jing, Chi, and Shen
Organ Meridians: Lungs, Kidneys, Heart, and Spleen
Spiritual Qualities: Calming, Opens the Heart Chakra, Love, Happiness, Peace of Mind, Lightness of Being, Uplifting—Allows the Spirit to Fly, Vitality, Lucid Dreaming, Good for those seeking Spiritual Attainment

Native to northern China and Korea, wild Asparagus Root is one of the most highly sought after herbs by monks, hermits, and holy people living in the mountainous regions of the Orient. The prized wild Asparagus Root was used by Daoists to open the heart chakra. A perfect Shen tonic, this herb stabilizes the emotional components of the heart, expanding one's view, creating a profound acceptance of things as they are, and allowing a natural flow of freedom, harmony, inner peace, and Universal love.

Most wild Asparagus Root found and available is yellow, wild red Asparagus Root is rare and quickly bought up, but both are good. Legends said that in Korea, where wild "red" Asparagus Root was more prevalent, Daoist hermits lived almost completely on this nutritious herb and after consuming it continuously, for long periods of time, developed the ability to fly. Asian sages claimed it was good for lucid dreaming and having dreams of flying. We believe that this is mainly referring to the ability of this precious root to uplift the human Spirit. This is the reason it is highly desirable for anyone seeking higher states of consciousness and enlightenment.

It is celebrated as one of the world's most prized Supertonic Herbs which nurtures all Three Treasures. Asparagus Root is noted for tonifying these major organs and energizing their meridians: Kidneys, Heart, Lungs, Spleen, and Stomach, helping to promote fluids. Its cooling nature moisturizes healthy tissue.

Asparagus Root is a superb Love tonic on all levels: physical, mental, and spiritual. Physically, it can strengthen those with sexual weakness if used for a prolonged period, by tonifying the Kidney yin. It is used to increase fertility and overcome impotence and frigidity. It increases sex drive, especially in women, by increasing fluids.

It is said to be a natural anti-depressant because it is uplifting to the emotions and mind.

Wild Asparagus Root is a significant Lung tonic; it moistens in a positive way and purifies the lungs, thereby improving all lung functions, and aids in breathing and removing toxins from the respiratory tract. It clears Lung heat while generating fluids and moistens dryness. Good for dry cough.

Consistent long-term consumption of this amazing root gives one the beauty of youth, including beautiful radiant skin that is soft, supple, and smooth; the result of the blood being purified and the lungs healthy.

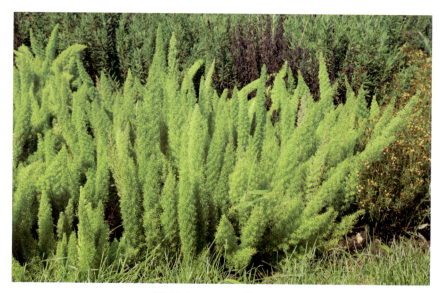

Wild Asparagus Growing

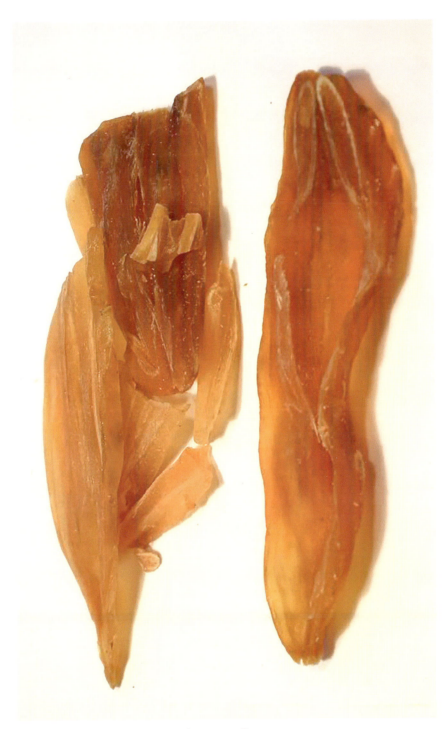

Asparagus Roots

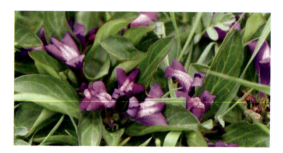
Polygala Plant with Flowers

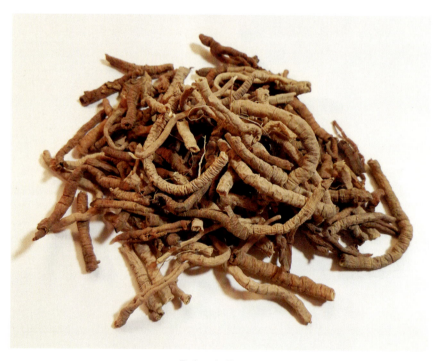
Polygala Roots

16. POLYGALA ROOT

Polygala Tenuifolia, Yuan Zhi

"The Will Strengthener"

Nourishes: Shen
Organ Meridians: Heart and Lungs
Spiritual Qualities: Clearing, Calming Emotions, Relaxing the Mind, Dreaming, Focus, Enhancing Creative Thinking and Visualization, Manifesting Power, Strengthens Willpower

Polygala is an incredibly empowering Shen tonic which has long been valued for its exceptional abilities to enhance one's Mind and Spirit. Daoists have widely used Polygala since ancient times as a tool for practitioners to overcome obstacles on the path to enlightenment. As a traditional Shen-stabilizing tonic, it is used to calm the emotions and relax the mind. But this potent root is said to affect mind in more empowering ways, as it contains what Daoists considered the Fourth Treasure, "Will."

To make progress on a spiritual path, any spiritual path, one must overcome challenges, face obstacles, find new solutions, and persevere to attain higher levels of conscious evolution. Polygala can help focus the mind and concentrate, a requirement for self-cultivation practices like meditation or other advanced spiritual practices. Traditionally, novice monks entering Chinese Daoist and Buddhist monasteries were given various herbal formulas to help them let go of old habits, energize them, and assist them in developing their new disciplines and challenges.

Interestingly, people have reported that consuming Polygala root enhanced their dreaming and creative thinking, manifesting new ideas and the way to turn our dreams into reality.

Daoists taught that creative visualization, "Yi," can actually become reality through "Will" power. Thus they taught that the will needed to be strengthened to cut through personal illusions to manifest our spiritual, physical, and worldly goals. Polygala became one of the most important herbs for Daoist practitioners and gained renown as the "Will Strengthener."

In this modern time, Polygala can be used by anyone who needs to strengthen the will to do and accomplish new things in their life. A useful aid in overcoming problems of drug abuse or any addiction: smoking, overeating, depression, or other compulsive thoughts and habits. We can all benefit from a stronger will to start new behaviors, new thinking patterns, new programs and projects; whatever it is we need to do to grow and become more complete individuals.

Polygala affects the Spirit in an extraordinary way that is unlike any other tonic or medicinal herbs. It connects the Kidney energy to the Heart energy, opening a special psychic channel that the Daoists call the Penetrating Vessel. Normally this Vessel is blocked internally and our sexual power and higher emotions and feeling of love can easily get derailed. Polygala uniquely connects the body and mind so that our sexuality connects with the feeling of love, giving us a deeper experience of unity, well-being, and happiness in life.

Contraindications: Use in moderation, especially in the beginning. It is often used to stabilize excessive dreaming, but in rare cases it increases the intensity of dreaming, for a short period of time.

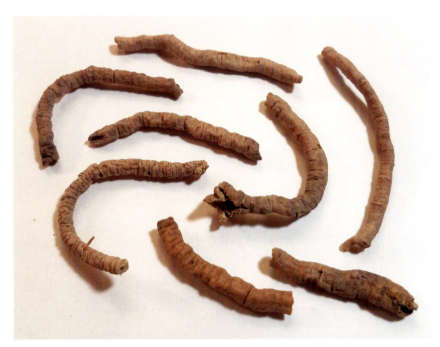

Polygala Roots

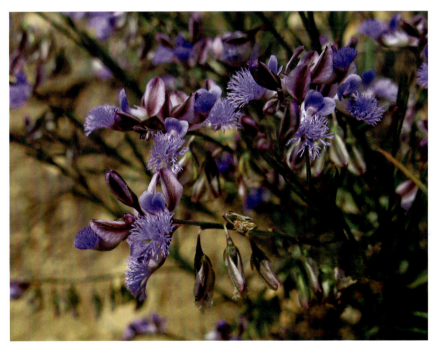

Polygala Flowers

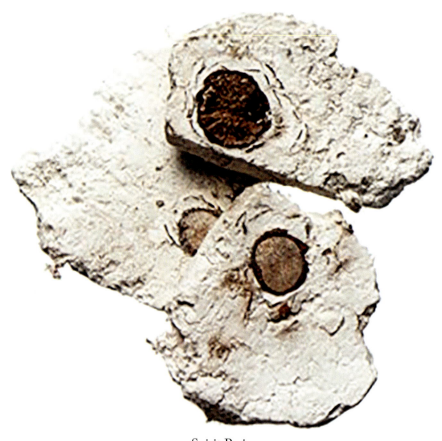

Spirit Poria

17. SPIRIT PORIA

Poria Cocos,
Fu Shen

Nourishes: Shen and Chi
Organ Meridians: Heart, Spleen, and Kidneys
Spiritual Qualities: Calming, Mental and Emotional Balance, Uplifting, Develops Spirit

Spirit Poria has been consumed by Daoists for centuries, and it is highly revered by spiritual seekers throughout Asia. The Daoists believe it possesses a special ability to lift the human spirit and develop Shen-Spirit. Spirit Poria has become known and respected as a supreme Shen tonic.

The Poria mushroom grows on the deep roots of pine trees. When the pine roots integrate into the solid fungal mass, the mycelium, and so contain the spirit of the tree, as well as the mushroom's energies, it becomes known as Spirit Poria, not just regular Poria. This central area where the roots of the host wood run into the mushroom's solid body is the part harvested and consumed. Each slice of Spirit Poria contains about 20% of the original integrated pine root. Both the energy and the chemistry of the wood is also changed by the mushroom and is no longer just a pine root.

Daoist hermits have been known to live on this mushroom, using it as a primary food source. But more than just nutrition, Spirit Poria has the power to balance the emotions and calm the heart and the mind, which sets the foundation for meditation, spiritual cultivation, and personal transformation. Daoist sages and adepts used this special mushroom to help bring about enlightenment.

It can also be used as a Chi tonic to revitalize the whole being and bring long life. Traditional Chinese medicine uses it for treating fear, worry, and anxiety, essentially balancing and stabilizing the emotions. Spirit Poria is strengthening to the functions of the Heart, Spleen, and Kidneys. It has a long history of treating insomnia and cardiac imbalances, including heart palpitations. Spirit Poria also contains the beneficial qualities of regular Poria (Fu Ling), to move water (mildly diuretic), clear dampness, and tonify the immune system functions. Regular Poria is mainly used as Chi tonic to benefit the internal organs.

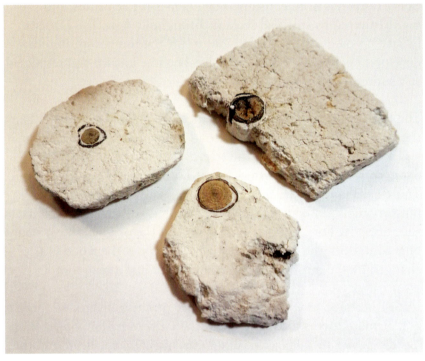

Spirit Poria
Note the woody center.
Spirit Poria grows on the roots of old pine trees and surrounds the root.

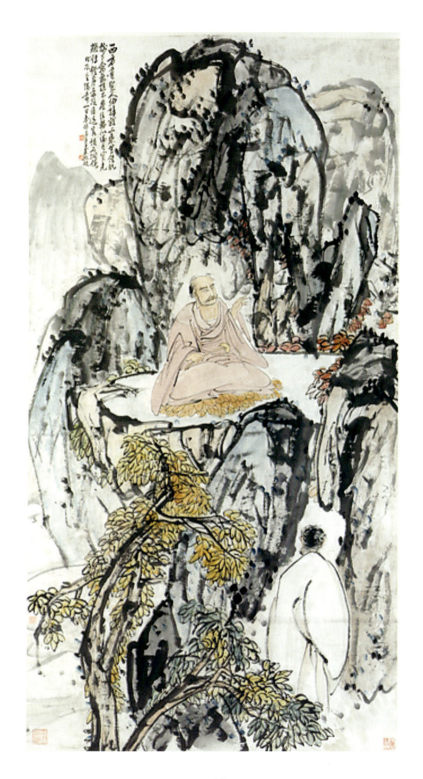

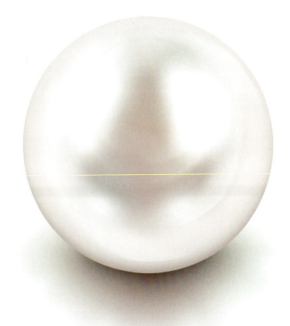

Natural Pearl

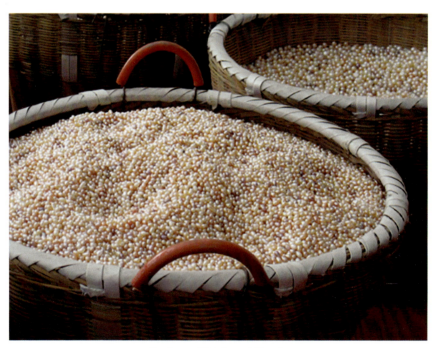

Baskets of Cultured Pearls

18. PEARL

Pteria Margaritifera, Zhen Zhu

Natural and Cultured

Nourishes: Shen
Organ Meridians: Heart and Liver
Spiritual Qualities: Energy, Vitality, Endurance, Restorative, Youthfulness, Beauty, Calmness

Pearl is held in high esteem as a Beauty tonic and a Shen tonic. It is certainly one of the best-kept beauty secrets of beautiful Asian women. It promotes regeneration of new skin cells, clears toxins, healing blemishes, discoloration, developing fine smooth texture and beautiful skin. A natural antioxidant, Pearl can assist in preventing skin from sagging and wrinkling. Continuous and consistent use can slow down the aging process of skin.

It can be taken internally as a tonic of hydrolyzed Pearl or applied externally as a cream.

A tonic gem, Pearl is a strong Shen stabilizer, composed of nutritional minerals and amino acids. Hydrolyzing the Pearl into a fine powder increases its ability to be absorbed by the body. The heart-soothing Pearl is used to relieve uneasiness of the mind and heart, slowing down nervousness and anxiety, and soothing tension. It prevents nerve weakness and disorders. Pearl is used to subdue fatigue and promote sound sleep; prolonged use will maintain vitality and energy and increase endurance.

Recently medical researchers have found many amazing uses for Pearl that you probably haven't heard of before. It relieves "wandering arthritis," internal fever, habitual constipation, and lowers blood pressure. It is said to improve muscle development and invigorate blood circulation. It is of benefit in reproduction and can heal inflammation of the uterus.

The precious Pearl is a boon for vision; it can remove visual obstacles and improve eyesight.

Studies have also shown that hydrolyzed Pearl can prevent osteoporosis and cardiovascular disease.

Another find that will make mothers happy: hydrolyzed Pearl powder can promote the growth of children's teeth and bones, and even improve the growing child's intelligence.

Natural pearls are by far the best quality for tonics, but they are extremely expensive and are often mixed with the powder of cultured (cultivated) pearls.

Contraindications: None. It is extremely safe and can be used throughout one's lifetime without negative side effects. Do not use pearls unless they are or can be hydrolyzed and obtained from reliable sources.

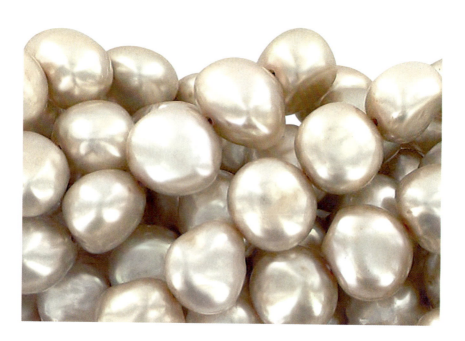

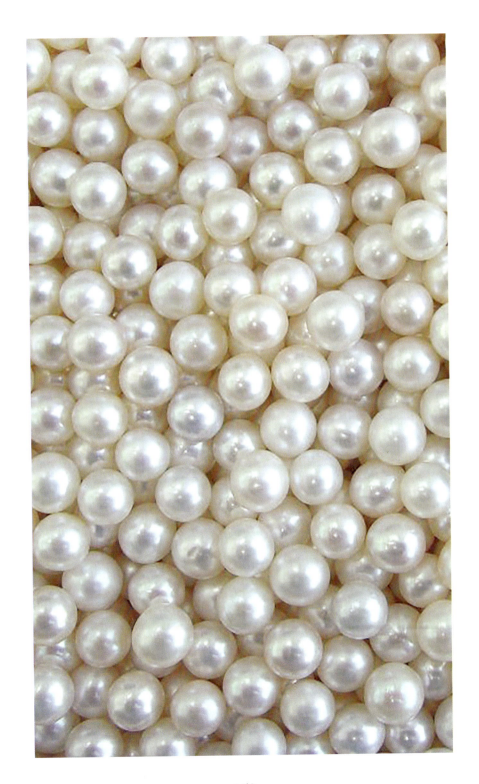

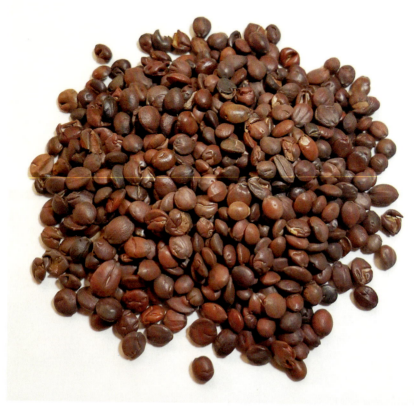

Zizyphus Seeds

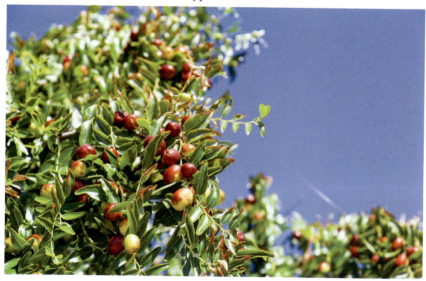

Jujube Dates (Zizyphus)

19. ZIZYPHUS SEED

Zizyphus Spinosa Hu, Zizyphus Sativa, Suan Zao Ren

"Calm the Heart Seed"

Nourishes: Blood and Shen
Organ Meridians: Heart and Liver
Spiritual Qualities: Relieving, Revitalizing, Returning to Balance, Calm Spirit, Tranquility

Zizyphus seed is the primary substance of sedative formulas in Tonic Herbalism. It makes the patient's mind calm and tranquil. Zizyphus spinosa is the seed of the wild Jujube date, a sweet red date native to southern Asia, especially China, Korea, and India. Now it is cultivated worldwide.

Shennong describes Zizyphus in the *Shennong Bencao Jing*: "Zizyphus is sour and balanced (in nature; being neither too warming or cooling, but combining both warming and cooling effects). It mainly treats heart and abdominal cold and heat and evil binding Chi, aching, pain in the limbs, and damp impediment. Protracted taking may quiet the five viscera, make the body light, and prolong life. It grows in rivers and swamps."

This calming seed is used in Heart-Blood tonics, as well as most sedative tonics. Zizyphus seed is gentle, mild, and effective. It has a slightly hypnotic effect on the mind. It is good for treating nervous individuals because it quiets anxiety and overthinking. It is both nourishing and revitalizing to those weakened by the fight-or-flight response. Zizyphus distinctly relieves people suffering from restless sleep, excessive dreaming, nightmares, or insomnia due to stress. Take as an evening tea before bed, for a good nights sleep. Traditionally it has been called the "Calm the Heart Seed." The Heart is the center of Shen. Zizyphus seed has a stabilizing effect on Shen by calming emotions, despair, and hurt feelings. It is especially effective when used with other Shen-stabilizing Tonic Herbs. It nourishes Yin. Scientific research has show that it can be used to prevent or benefit arrhythmia or heart palpitations. It is also used as a treatment for anemia.

The seed, when fried first and then cooled as a preparation, is known to be useful for nourishing the Liver blood. The raw herb may be used to drain the Liver and gallbladder. The roasted seed extract can be used to avoid the hypnotic affect. Both raw and prepared seeds have similar sedative abilities and calm the spirit. The Zizyphus fruit, Jujube, may also be used in some formulas or teas. Jujube is an excellent Chi tonic that can replenish Chi in the spleen and stomach, strengthen muscles, and nourish the Blood. It is also a mild Shen tonic that calms the mind, providing energy without causing any drowsiness.

Contraindications: Be prepared, it many cause drowsiness. Avoid using when you have diarrhea.

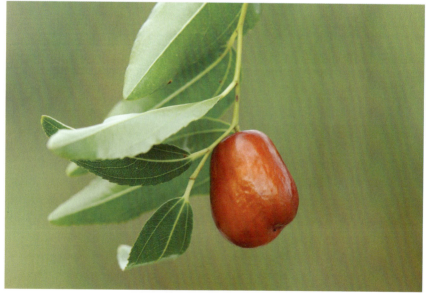

Jujube

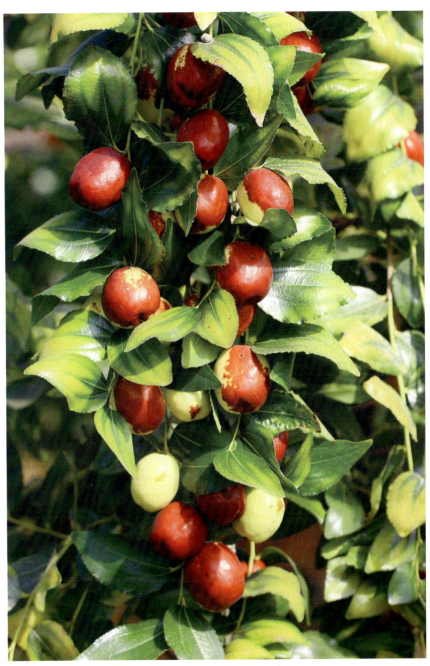
Jujube (Zizyphus) Tree

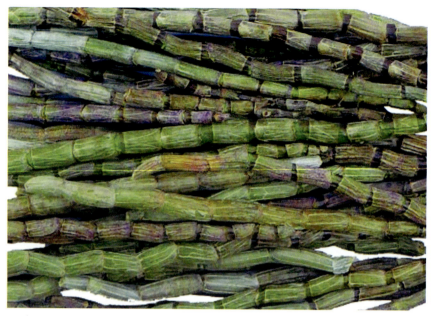

Dendrobium Stems

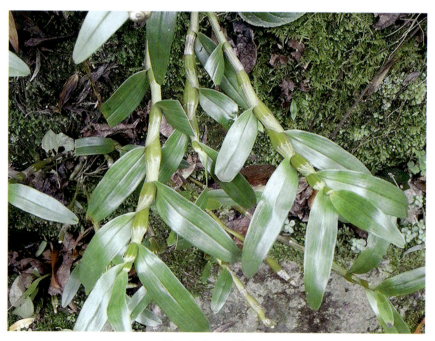

Dendrobium Plants

20. DENDROBIUM

Dendrobium Nobile, Shi Hu, Suk Gok

"The Healer's Tea"

Nourishes: Yin Jing
Organ Meridians: Kidneys, Lungs, and Stomach
Spiritual Qualities: Healing Energy, Rejuvenation, Longevity

The stem and leaves of the beautiful Chinese orchid, Dendrobium Nobile, make an excellent Yin Jing tonic used in the Orient for centuries. Taoists will tell you the real potency of the orchid is in its flower pod. Dendrobium is renowned as a restorative Jing tonic. It can quickly replace spent Jing essence and build adaptogenic power. The Kidneys serve as the body's reservoir of Jing. Dendrobium is a longevity promoting herb which nourishes the Kidneys, Lungs, and Stomach and also tastes delicious. It was extensively used by Daoist hermits and sages, who considered it so beneficial they would drink it daily.

Known as the Healer's Tea, it is an important herb for people working as healers, who especially use energy and hands-on techniques. This healing orchid plant is said to provide healing energy to the body of the Healer which can then be transmitted to others, as well as replacing spent healing energy. It is a God-send for body workers, massage therapists, and those who are giving, from a deep level of themselves, energy to others. Master Sung Jin Park drank this simple tea daily for many years.

In China it is mainly used now to replenish body fluids exhausted from hot dry conditions. As a Yin Tonic that moistens both the Stomach and the Lungs, Dendrobium nourishes the saliva and effectively treats dryness issues such as dry mouth, thirst, and mouth sores, cough, and sunstroke. Also it treats breathing and lung issues by moistening the lungs and air passages affected by air pollution, dry weather, or smoke.

Asian women love Dendrobium's capacity for promoting moist skin and beautiful complexions when drinking it consistently.

The Denbrobium orchid stem is an excellent longevity herb. It is widely used in the Orient with a small amount of Licorice. This is called the Honeymooners' Tea, for those who engage in an over abundance of sexual activity and are in need of restoring their spent energy and lost fluids.

Contraindications: Safe as a tonic herb. Use in moderation. Avoid use during early symptoms of fever and phlegm accumulation.

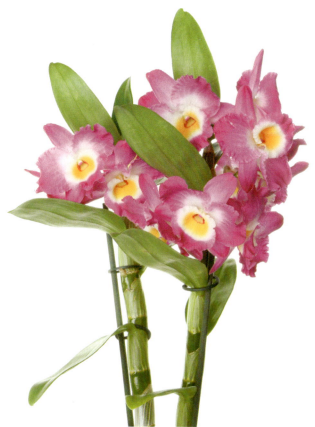

Dendrobium Nobile Orchids

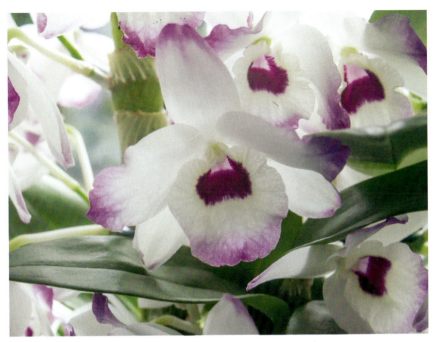

Dendrobium Nobile Orchids

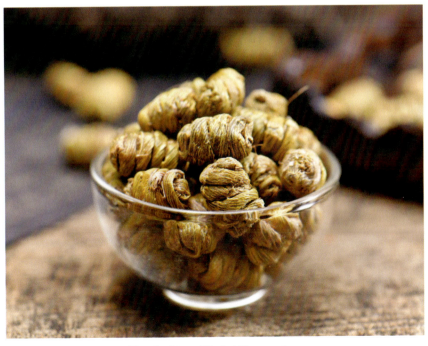

Dendrobium Herbal Preparation

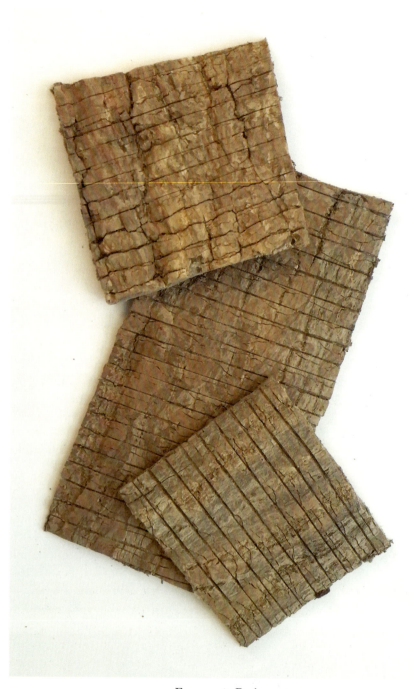

Eucommia Bark

21. EUCOMMIA BARK

Eucommia Ulmoides, Du Zhong

Nourishes: Yang Jing and Yin Jing
Organ Meridians: Kidneys and Liver
Spiritual Qualities: Relief, Balances, Calms, Restorative, Strengthening

Eucommia bark produces a superlative Yin and Yang tonic renowned for nourishing and tonifying the Kidneys' functions. Shennong wrote about Eucommia as the second entry in the first recorded Chinese herbal pharmacopoeia, *The Divine Farmer's Materia Medica,* around 2,500 years ago.

Eucommia's tonifying power makes it the primary herb used to strengthen the skeletal structure. This legendary bark promotes healthy skeletal growth and builds strong, sturdy, and flexible bones. Eucommia similarly strengthens the muscles, ligaments, tendons, and joints that support the bones. It is used to help heal and mend broken bones and tissues, no matter what age.

Eucommia is one of the few Tonic Herbs that can be used alone but is generally combined with other herbs which can build balanced powerful Kidney Yin and Yang. It is specifically used to relieve lower back and knee problems where there is stiffness, swelling, dislocation, pain, or weakness.

This herb has varying degrees of regulation on the immune system, endocrine system, central nervous system, circulatory system, and urinary systems. What's more, it can excite the hypothalamus-pituitary-adrenal cortex system and strengthen the adrenal function. Called Du Zhong in China, it is said to strengthen the entire body, the endocrine system, and sexual functions. Kidney Jing is a important factor in conception. Eucommia is a foremost component of tonics designed for those wanting to conceive a child. Eucommia is a prime herb to enhance and promote both female fertility and male potency.

For thousands of years, Eucommia has been used to treat hypertension and high blood pressure symptoms. More recent studies in the West support the traditional functions of Eucommia. Western Research has proven that both the bark and leaves have hypotensive action, lowering blood pressure over a period of consistent use. Furthermore, studies support that it provides phagocytic and immunological activity in the human body when combined with other herbs such as Astragalus and Codonopsis. This potent bark is mildly sedative, anti-inflammatory, and diuretic.

Chinese medical scholar and herbalist Li Shizhen wrote the *Compendium of Materia Medica, Bencao Gangmu*, in 1596. His book took 27 years to complete and is considered the greatest scientific achievement of the Ming Dynasty era, and became a standard reference text for natural medicine. Li Shizhen tells that the Chinese name for Eucommia revolved around an old story, "At one time there was a man named Du Zhong who took this herb and became enlightened; therefore, it was named after him."

Safe and mild. Native to Central and Eastern China.

Contraindications: None

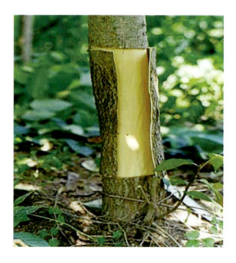

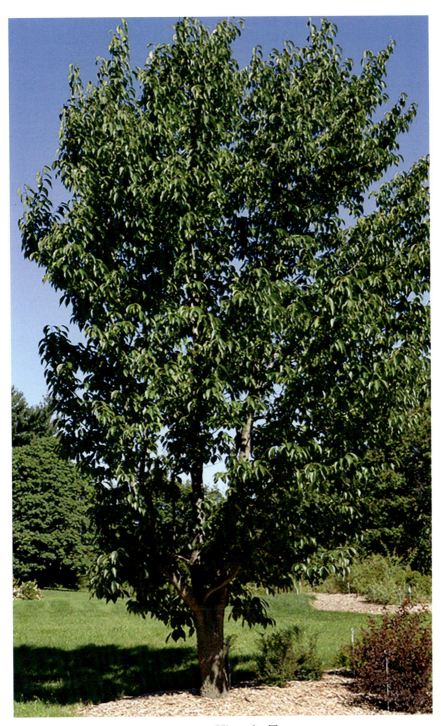
Eucommia Ulmoides Tree

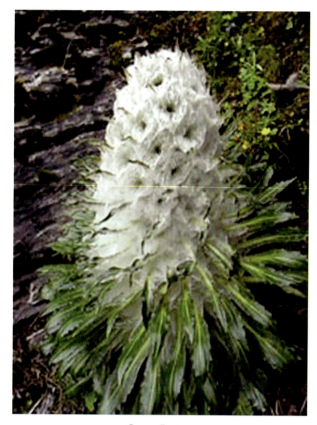

Snow Lotus

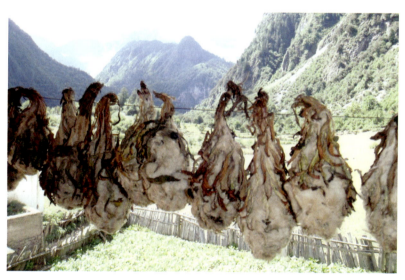

Snow Lotus Drying

22. SNOW LOTUS

Saussurea Involucrate, Saussurea Laniceps, Xue Lian, Tian Shan Xue Lian

A Supporting Herb: Adaptogen and Cleansing tonic
Spiritual Qualities: Clearing, Strengthening, Calmness, Beauty

Rarest of rare, this magnificent cottony, pure white flower, the Snow Lotus, grows wild well beyond 18,000 feet, above the snowline in the highest of the Himalayan mountains. In ancient times, if you were going to see the Empress in China, you would be wise to take Snow Lotus as a gift, the supreme beauty tonic desired by the Asian woman. Growing on steep and unstable sheer mountain slopes, acquiring this herb is not an easy task. The plant grows slowly for seven to ten years. The entire plant is used for medicinal purposes. Being extremely rare indeed, this precious flower blooms but once every five years. It is one of the three tonic herbal treasures of the Himalayan region used in both Chinese and Tibetan Medicine. In China and Tibet there are actually twelve types of Saussurea historically grown wild and used in Chinese medicine.

Snow Lotus is a wonderful tonic that enhances beauty, along with promoting radiant skin, one reason it is so loved by women. Combining it with Pearl Powder, Goji Berries, and Logan Fruit enhances the effects, creating firm, moist skin that is smooth, soft, and beautiful.

Containing many medicinal benefits, it is a profound adaptogen renowned for its detoxifying properties. It is a suburb cleansing tonic that is effective against radiation, as well as other health issues. It is known to be supportive and effective in treating weakness, muscle soreness, rheumatism, headache, high blood pressure, arthritis, and lumbago. It assists in alleviating women of irregular menstruation. (menorrhagia) and impotence.

INDEX

Note: Page numbers in **bold** indicate the pages for a main entry on the specific tonic herb

Adrenal glands, 55, 98, 125
Albizzia, 34, 54, **142–143**
America Ginseng, **110–111**
The Ancient Wisdom of Chinese Tonic Herbs (Teeguarden), 54
"The Anti-Aging Herbs of China" Xiao Pei-Gen, 32–33
Asparagus Root, 34
Astragalus, 115, **138–141**, 170

Back, lower, 121, 125, 169
Beauty tonic, 32, 99, 157, 173
Beckwith, Rev. Michael, 66, 72
Beijing Medicinal Plant Garden, 68–69
Blood tonic, 99, 125, 129, 135, 139, 161
Bodhidharma (Indian Buddhist monk), 72–74, 78–79
Bones, 55, 158, 169
Brain tonic, 99, 114, 117, 118
Buddha Nature, 72
Buddhism, 9, 40, 57–58, 79

Carradine, David, 70–71
Chaga, 79, **130–133**
Changbai Mountain, 48–52
    description, 49
    expedition to, 36, 48–52
    Ginseng farms, 49
    Ginseng Gardens, 46

Heaven Lake, vi, 48–49, 51
Reishi farms, 48, 49, 51–52
Wild Reishi from, 32
Changbaishan National Nature Reserve, 49
Chi (Qi), 19–21, 27, 29, 31, 35, 54, 75. *See also* specific herbs
Chi tonics, 20, 35, 108, 111, 129, 132, 153, 154, 162
China trips, 38–45, 48–52
    Changbai Mountain, 46, 48–52
    herb market, 43–45
    Institute of Medicinal Plant Development, 68
    Medicinal Plant Garden, 68–69
    Shaolin Temple pilgrimage, 70–80
    White Cloud Temple, 67–68
Compendium of Materia Medica (Bencao Gangmu) (Li Shizhen), 23
Concentration, 92, 97, 99, 102
Confucianism, 40
Cordyceps, 32, 55, **120–123**
Cousens, Gabriel, 66, 69, 72

Dao De Ching (Lao Tzu), 71
Daoism, 9, 36, 40, 72
Daoist longevity techniques, 27–31, 77

Daoist mountain hermits, 25–28
Dendrobium, **164–167**
Di Dao, Di Dao herbs, 46–47
Dragon Herbs (company), 32, 33, 34, 47, 52, 85–86
Duanwood Reishi, 35, 51–52, 90, 94

8 Immortals tincture, 35
Eight Silken Brocades (Baduanjin), 30–31, 77
Elixir Bar, 34–37
Endurance
  Astragalus for, 139
  Cordyceps for, 55
  Ginseng for, 102, 107–108, 111
  Pearl for, 157
  Rhodiola for, 117
  Schizandra for, 99
Eucommia Bark, **168–171**
Eyes/vision, 55, 154

FITT™ (Fingerprint Identical Transfer Technology), 33

Gallbladder, 162
Ginseng (Panax Ginseng), 4, 44–45, **100–104**. *See also* America Ginseng; Siberian Ginseng
Glands, 98, 125
Goddess Magu, 5, 7, 48, 50
Goji Berries. *See* Lycium Fruit (Goji Berries)
Gracie family, 54–55
Grandfather Cachora (Yaqui Indian shaman), 55–57

Gynostemma, **112–114**, 115
He Shou Wu (Polygonum), 12–13
Heart
  Albizzia for, 143
  Cordyceps for, 122
  Ginseng root for, 102
  Goji berries for, 136
  Gynostemma for, 113
  Pearl for, 157
  Polygala root for, 149–150
  Rehmannia root for, 129
  Reishi for, 91–93
  Rhodiola for, 118
  Schizandra berries for, 97–98
  Siberian Ginseng for, 107
  Spirit Poria for, 153–154
  Wild Asparagus root for, 144–146
  Zizyphus seed for, 161–162
Heart-blood tonics, 161
Heaven Lake (Changbai Mountain), 48–49, 51
Heaven Mountain (China), 42, 47, 86, 136
Heaven Mountain® Goji Berries, 42, 47
Herb market (China), 43–45
Hinduism, 9, 72

I-Ching, 11
India, viii, 55, 59–66, 72
Institute of Medicinal Plant Development (IMPLAD; Beijing), 68
Intelligence, 99, 117, 158
Intestines, 140

The Jade Emperor's Mind Seal Classic: A Taoist Guide to Health, Longevity, and Immortality (Olson), 20–21
Jiao Gu Lan. *See* Gynostemma
Jing, 18–21, 26, 29, 54, 91. *See also* specific herbs
Joints, 169
Jujube. *See* Zizyphus Seeds

Kaya Kalpa (herbal formula), 63–65
Kidney tonic, 98, 99, 132
Kidney Yin tonic, 145
Kung Fu (martial art), 71, 73, 74, 77, 79
"Kung Fu" TV show, 70–72

Lao Tzu, 71, 72
Li Qing Yun (herbalist), 82–83
Li Shizhen (herbalist), 23–24
Ligaments, 55, 169
Liver
    Albizzia for, 143
    Chaga for, 131–132
    Eucommia bark for, 169
    Goji berries for, 136
    Gynostemma for, 113–114
    Lyceum fruit for, 135
    Pearl for, 157
    Polygonum for, 125
    Rehmannia Root for, 129
    Reishi for, 91–93
    Schizandra berries for, 97–99
    Siberian Ginseng for, 107–108
    Zizyphus seed for, 161–162
Liver tonic, 98, 99, 132

Longevity tonic, 91, 99, 122, 145–146
Love tonic, 146
Lu Zi, 21
Lung tonic, 122, 145–146
Lungs
    American Ginseng for, 111
    Astragalus for, 139
    Chaga for, 131–132
    Cordyceps for, 121–122
    Dendrobium for, 165
    Ginseng for, 101
    Goji berries for, 136
    Gynostemma for, 113
    Lycium fruit for, 135
    Polygala Root for, 149
    Reishi for, 91–92
    Schizandra berries for, 97–98
    Siberian Ginseng for, 107
    Wild Asparagus Root for, 145–146
Lycium Fruit (Goji Berries), 34, 42, 47, 82, 86, 134–137, 173

Mahasiddhas (Great Siddhas), 62
Man and Biosphere Program (UNESCO), 49
Memory, 99
Mind
    Cordyceps for, 121
    Ginseng root for, 102–103
    Gynostemma for, 114
    Pearl for, 157
    Polygala Root for, 149–150
    Reishi for, 92
    Schizandra berries for, 99
    Spirit Poria for, 153

Wild Asparagus Root for, 144–146
Zizyphus seed for, 161–162
Mind tonic, 99
Moo San Do Sha, 15, 17, 25–26, 28, 82, 125
Murty, T.S. Anantha, 62
Muscles, 55, 169

Nerves, 92, 100, 107, 114, 126

Pearl, **156–159**, 173
Polygala Root, **148–151**
Polygonum (He Shou Wu), 12, **124–127**

Qi. *See* Chi

Radiant Health, 6, 18, 23, 35, 44, 82–83, 182
Rehmannia Root, **128–129**
Reishi Mushroom, 4–5, 34, 48, 49, 79, 90–95. *See also* Duanwood Reishi
Rhodiola, 32, 54, **116–119**, 121
Rooted in Spirit: The Heart of Chinese Medicine, 11

Schizandra Berries, 20, 26, 29, 34, 50, 86, **96–99**, 115
Sex tonic, 99, 102, 121, 126, 129, 137
Shang Dynasty, 22
Shaolin Temple (China), 29–31, 70–80
Shen, 18, 20–21, 26, 29, 35, 54
Shen tonics, 91, 94–95, 99, 132, 143, 145, 149, 153, 157, 162. *See also* Reishi Mushroom

Shénnóng Běn Cao Jīng (Shennong's Materia Medica) (Shennong), 22–23
Shennong (herbalist), 22–23, 94, 100, 132, 161, 169
Shifu Shi Yan Zhuang, 77
Siberian Ginseng, **106–109**, 115
Siddha tradition, 60–62
Snow Lotus, 32, **172–173**
Spirit Poria, 54, **152–154**
Spiritual development, 81–84
Spleen
American Ginseng for, 111
Astragalus for, 139
Chaga for, 131–132
Ginseng for, 101
Gynostemma for, 113
Jujube for, 162
Schizandra berries for, 98
Siberian Ginseng for, 107–108
Spirit Poria for, 153–154
Wild Asparagus Root for, 145–146
Spring Dragon Longevity Tea, 86, 115
Stomach
American Ginseng for, 111
Asparagus Root for, 146
Astragalus Root for, 140
Chaga for, 132
Dendrobium for, 165
Jujube for, 162
Stress
Chaga for reducing, 132
Ginseng root for reducing, 102–103
Reishi for reducing, 91–93

Siberian Ginseng for reducing, 107
Sun Si-Miao (master herbalist), 135
Sung Jin Park, ix, 15–17, 25, 28–29, 50, 97, 125, 165
Superior Herbs, 23

Tao Hong-Jing (master herbalist), 135
Taoism. *See* Daoism
Tapaswiji Maharaj (Mahasiddha), 62–64, 65
Teeth, 158
Tendons, 55, 125, 169
Three Treasures Philosophy, 18–21. *See also* Chi; Jing; Shen
Tibetan Buddhism, 9, 57–58, 59
Tonic Herbs/Herbalism. *See also* specific tonic herbs
   description, viii, 6
   growth of in America, 14–17
   history of, 22–24
   instructions for taking, 85–87
   Teeguarden's discovery of, ix, 12–13
"Tortoise-Sparrow-Dog" article *(Time)*, 82
Traditional Chinese Medicine (TCM), 22–24
Tree of Life Healing Center, 66

Weight-Loss Herb. *See* Gynostemma
Wild Asparagus Root, 54, **144–147**
Wild Reishi, 32, 54

Xiao Pei-Gen, 32–33

Yang Jing tonics, 121, 135, 169
Yang tonic, 99, 169
Yin Jing tonics, 121, 125, 129, 135, 145, 165, 169
Yin tonic, 99, 145, 165
Yin/Yang balance, 10

Zen Buddhism, 72, 79
Zizyphus Seeds, **160–163**

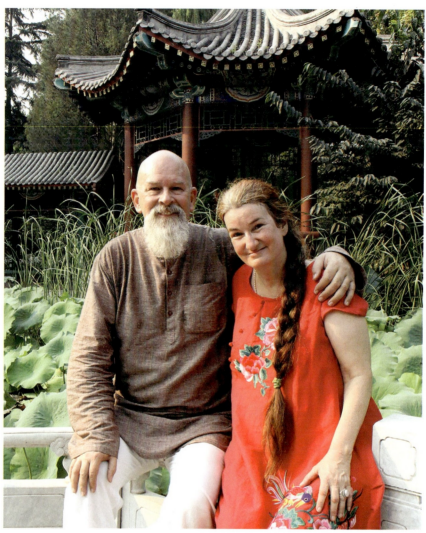

It is our sincere wish that everyone who reads this book finds within it inspiration to attain Radiant Health and full Enlightenment.
Love and Light,
Ganga and Tara